# *TOXIC TEETH*

How a Biological (Holistic) Dentist Can Help You Cure Cancer, Facial Pain, Autoimmune, Heart, and Other Disease Caused By Infected Gums, Root Canals, Jawbone Cavitations, and Toxic Metals

*Y.L. Wright, M.A.*

and

*J.M. Swartz, M.D.*

Copyright © 2016 by Y.L. Wright M.A. and J.M. Swartz M.D.
ISBN 978-1-365-31638-8
Lulu Press, Inc.

All Rights Reserved. No part of this document may be reproduced without written consent from the authors.

**MEDICAL DISCLAIMER:**
The following text contains the opinions and ideas of the authors. Careful attention has been paid to insure the accuracy of the information, but the authors and the publisher cannot assume responsibility for the validity or consequences of its use. This information is not intended to diagnose or treat any disease. We are only providing education and our point of view. The authors are not rendering medical, health, or any other professional services. See your medical or health professional concerning any health concerns or before following any suggestions made in this book or drawing inferences from it. The authors specifically disclaim all responsibility for any liability, loss, or risk incurred as a direct or indirect consequence of using this book's contents. Any use of the information found in this book is the sole responsibility of the reader. Any suggestions found in this book are to be followed only under the supervision of a medical doctor and/or a trained dentist.

**DEDICATION:**
"Toxic Teeth" is written for you. If even one person finds their way out of chronic disease and suffering into health, it has been worth it. Read this book and learn how to avoid and reverse the development of systemic disease that may begin from problems in your mouth.

**OTHER BOOKS BY Y.L. WRIGHT, M.A. AND J.M. SWARTZ, M.D.:**
**"MEN'S HORMONES MADE EASY! How to Treat: Low Testosterone, Low Growth Hormone, Erectile Dysfunction, BPH, Andropause, Insulin Resistance, Adrenal Fatigue, Thyroid, Osteoporosis, High Estrogen, and DHT!"** Prevent and Reverse: Manopause, Prostate Issues, Heart Disease, and Cancer. *See how hormone issues at any age may:* Wreck your relationship. Make you fat. Accelerate aging and death. *Learn how to SAFELY:* Improve your sexual performance. Increase your energy, motivation, and sex drive. Strengthen muscles and bones. This book is designed to be a workbook in anti-aging medicine for self-responsible men who want to intelligently work with their physicians for optimal life and longevity. It is also an update on the diagnosis and treatment of mild, moderate, and severe hormonal problems for physicians who have been unable to keep up-to-date on anti-aging medicine.

**"Bioidentical Hormones Made Easy!"** Learn about bioidentical hormone replacement therapy (BHRT) for women in a quick and easy book.

**"Secrets about Growth Hormone to Build Muscle, Increase Bone Density, and Burn Body Fat!"** See how Growth Hormone levels drop as we get older, when to intervene, and what treatment options are available to optimize health.

**"Secrets about Bioidentical Hormones to Lose Fat and Prevent Cancer, Heart Disease, Menopause, and Andropause by Optimizing Adrenals, Thyroid, Estrogen, Progesterone, Testosterone, and Growth Hormone!"** Learn about the leading edge of anti-aging medicine--Bioidentical Hormone Therapy. Discover how to diagnose hormonal abnormalities. You will also be given treatment options. Learn how hormones become unbalanced, especially during menopause and andropause.

**"Fat Loss Secrets that Really Work--Balance Your Hormones: Insulin, Estrogen, Progesterone, Testosterone, Thyroid, Cortisol, and DHEA!"** Find out exactly how to correct the hormonal problems that prevent you from losing fat, especially belly fat, and how to normalize your weight for the rest of your life.

**"Secrets about the HCG Diet! Treatment Guide, Controversy, Benefits, Risks, Side Effects, and Contraindications."** Discover the answers to: What is hCG? How does hCG work? How is it used in a program to lose weight?

**"SECRETS to LOSE TOXIC BELLY FAT! Heal Your Sick Metabolism Using State-Of-The-Art Medical Testing and Treatment With Detoxification, Diet, Lifestyle, Supplements, and Bioidentical Hormones."** Toxic belly fat is a parasite that preserves itself at the expense of its host -- YOU! Lose toxic belly fat and regain metabolic health by correcting the sick metabolism associated with toxic belly fat.

**"The Wisdom of Bioidentical Hormones In Menopause, Perimenopause, and Premenopause! Unleash the power of Estrogen, Progesterone, Testosterone, Cortisol, DHEA, Growth Hormone, Pregnenolone, Oxytocin, Vitamin D3, and Melatonin!"** THE WISDOM OF BIOIDENTICAL HORMONES lies in knowing when and how to use them. This book can help you determine which methods of bioidentical hormone replacement therapy (BHRT), if any, may work best for YOU, no matter how old you are, whether you are in menopause, perimenopause, or even younger. To really feel at your best, you may or may not need bioidentical hormone replacement. Are bioidentical hormones safe? Do they cause cancer? Are there side effects? When should you begin to use them? What tests are needed? How can you find a doctor who will prescribe the bioidentical hormones that will work best for you? Get this book and learn the answers to all of these questions.

# CONTENTS

1. TOXIC TEETH ARE MAKING US SICK. .................5
2. LUPUS, MENTAL ILLNESS, CANCER GONE. ......6
3. MY DENTAL DECEPTION AND HEALING. .........10
4. DISEASES CAUSED BY MOUTH PROBLEMS. ..21
5. CHOOSE YOUR DENTIST WISELY! ....................25
6. DENTAL TOXINS. ................................................32
7. GUM DISEASE. ....................................................43
8. ROOT CANALS: SOURCES OF INFECTION.......50
9. JAWBONE CAVITATIONS......................................54
10. PROBLEMS WITH WISDOM TEETH. ..................67
11. PROGRESSIVE DENTAL THERAPIES. .............69
12. LEAKY GUT AND ORAL HEALTH. .....................71
13. HEAL WITH ESSENTIAL OILS. ..........................73
14. CONCLUSION. ....................................................75
REFERENCES. ........................................................76

## 1. TOXIC TEETH ARE MAKING US SICK.

**BEFORE YOU DECIDE TO BUY A HORSE, IT IS A GOOD IDEA TO LOOK INSIDE ITS MOUTH.** To find out how healthy the horse is, pull back the horse's lips and examine the gums and teeth thoroughly. It is the same with you and me. Our own health is directly affected by dental issues. Sneaky and often silent, many dental issues may go undiagnosed for years, if ever.

- Toxic heavy metals used in fillings, crowns, bridges, partials, dentures, and implants continually seep into every cell in our bodies creating heavy metal poisoning that triggers disease.[1]
- Whether or not we know it, over half of us harbor gum infections.[2]
- If we have ever had teeth extracted, it is quite likely that cesspools of infection (cavitations)[3] bubble deep within our jawbones.[4]
- Root canal teeth seed nasty infections, causing untold suffering.[5,6]

**I am one of the lucky ones.** I recently uncovered many horrific, yet silent, dental issues and corrected them. This resulted in the disappearance of a nagging pain behind my eye and decreased autoimmune symptoms. The asthma, allergies, arthritis, poor digestion, and fatigue that had plagued me for decades are now gone.

**Most people aren't so fortunate.** Their undiagnosed dental problems may lead to diseases that incapacitate and eventually kill them. They don't know why they got sick. Their doctors tell them that the cause of their illness is unknown and that the only treatments are pills, needles, surgery, or radiation.

**Dental infections spread through the bloodstream** into our brains, hearts,[7] and other organs, leading to many kinds of diseases,[8] such as heart disease,[9,10] cancer,[11] autoimmune diseases (allergies, asthma, thyroid problems),[12] and facial pain,[13] although your doctor may not believe that. Your doctor needs to read this book.

**READ ON TO LEARN SECRETS ABOUT TOXIC TEETH unknown to most people, including most dentists.** Discover how to heal from disease-causing dental issues.
- **Gum disease.**
- **The toxicity from root canals.**
- **Jawbone disease--often silent.**
- **Toxic (incompatible to you) materials used in:**
    - **Fillings.**
    - **Implants.**
    - **Bridges.**
    - **Crowns.**
    - **Dentures.**

## 2. LUPUS, MENTAL ILLNESS, CANCER GONE.

To illustrate how dental issues can destroy your health and find out how to restore good health again, let's consider what happened to Samantha, Dr. Larry, and Julie.

- First let's see how Samantha became crippled with pain after getting two root canals. Then we will discover how she reversed her illness and got her health back.
- Then let's consider the predicament of Dr. Larry, a dentist who literally lost his mind after becoming poisoned by the mercury that he used to fill cavities. We will see how he recovered his sanity and improved the safety of his dental procedures.
- After that, we will discover how Julie got rid of a deadly breast cancer by following a complete detox program, which prioritized cleaning up all of the problems in her mouth.

### Samantha's root canals made her sick.

**Samantha was sparring in karate when she was kicked hard in the front teeth by an opponent's foot.** One of her front teeth died. In order to save the tooth from extraction, her dentist performed a root canal treatment on that tooth. About a year later, the tooth next to it died, and she got a root canal on that tooth, too.

Just three weeks after that second root canal was done, Samantha developed arthritis in her hands that was so bad that she could not work at her job as a massage therapist. The arthritis pain worsened, spreading to every joint in her body. Six months later she could not even get out of bed without help. Blood tests revealed the presence of an autoimmune disease called systemic lupus erythematosus (lupus). Her body was literally attacking itself. Inflammation was affecting her joints, skin, kidneys, blood cells, brain, heart, and lungs.

Samantha had a sneaking suspicion that the root canal treatments might have had something to do with this awful disease. As a result, she followed her intuition and decided to get those two front teeth that had the root canals removed. Within three weeks after the removal of the root canal teeth, 90% of her arthritis had vanished, and her lupus symptoms had completely disappeared. Her bloodwork now came back normal.

She joyfully leaped out of bed in the mornings, grateful to return to her work and an active life. With the removal of the root canals, the bacteria coming from the dead root-canal teeth also disappeared. These bacteria and their waste products had been carried by the bloodstream into her whole body. Without that continual bacterial seeding into the rest of her body, the inflammation subsided. When the inflammation subsided, she was able to heal from all of the lupus symptoms.

**The good news is that disease can be healed when you remove the underlying conditions that are contributing to that disease.** Sometimes, doing something that we have been led to believe is safe (like getting root canals) can be the impetus that pushes us over the edge of the cliff into ill health.

In Samantha's case, it was the second root canal that pushed her over that precipice into chronic disease. Her immune system could not cope with the huge onslaught of toxins produced by the bacteria in her root canals. Removing those root canals allowed her to return to health.

## Dr. Larry learns an important lesson.

**Dr. Larry was a dentist who was using amalgams without using a safe protocol.** Amalgams are the common silver, black, or gray fillings that have been placed into the teeth of millions of people. Amalgams consist of about half mercury and the rest other metals. They are not usually called mercury fillings, but are most often referred to as amalgams or silver fillings. Most people have no idea of the toxicity of these amalgams, and that they can lead to terrible health problems.

**Mercury is never safe, and therefore amalgams are never safe.** Mercury adversely affects everyone who gets it put into their mouths.

There are many factors that affect the type and severity of symptoms and length of time for symptoms to occur. Some people experience severe symptoms immediately. Others may only notice mild symptoms that may not appear for years. In any case, the connection between the mercury-laden fillings and health problems is rarely suspected.

Dr. Larry had never been aware of the dangers of mercury poisoning caused by the mercury that he was using in amalgam fillings. Dr. Larry had no idea that he was allowing his own office to become filled with toxic mercury vapors, poisoning himself, his patients, his staff, and anyone else who entered. His dental training and continuing education never mentioned anything about the toxicity of amalgam fillings. Just like all the other dental students before him and continuing to this day, Dr. Larry was never taught in dental school that both he and his patients were being poisoned by the mercury in the amalgams used to fill the cavities in their teeth. By accepting what he was taught in dental school (that mercury in the mouth is not a problem), Dr. Larry had unwittingly intoxicated himself and his patients with the mercury that he was placing and extracting.

Dr. Larry eventually became terribly depressed and confused from the mercury poisoning his brain. Mercury poisoning has devastating effects on cognition and mood.[14] His volatile temper had caused most of his staff to quit their jobs. At the insistence of his family, he checked himself in to a mental health facility. After staying in the mental health facility for a few weeks and being out of the toxic environment of his dental office, he detoxed enough of the mercury out of his system to get his wits about him.

A friend mentioned to him that he might have mercury toxicity. A heavy metals test confirmed that Dr. Larry did indeed have very high levels of this toxic heavy metal. Dr. Larry began to research the facts about mercury poisoning and discovered that dentists and other dental professionals who are exposed to mercury have significantly more mental and neurological problems,[15] a higher rate of suicide,[16] more respiratory problems,[17] and more cardiovascular problems[18] than average. As he placed and removed the mercury fillings without proper safety protocols, everyone in the office breathed the mercury vapors that permeated the air.[19] Dr. Larry had no system for safely disposing of the solid mercury waste, either. Some went down the drain. Some went into the trash that was thrown into a truck and dumped into the landfill. Some fell onto people's clothes. Some dropped onto the carpets and then were tracked into people's homes.

After he left the mental health facility, Dr. Larry became a believer in strict protocols for removing mercury fillings safely. Dr. Larry enrolled in a training course to learn how to safely remove amalgams and received certification from the International Academy of Oral Medicine and Toxicology[20] (IAOMT) to prove his newfound competence. He bought special equipment to remove the mercury fillings safely. He installed mercury amalgam separators, serviced by a hazardous waste removal company.

**Dr. Larry knew that he had to work hard and work for the rest of his life to detoxify the mercury that had been deposited into the tissues all over his body.** He bought an inexpensive far infrared sauna and sweated in his detox box for at least an hour every day. He also received regular intravenous chelation treatments from his physician. In addition, he carefully watched his diet to avoid eating foods that are known to be high in mercury (particularly tuna fish).

## How Julie got rid of a deadly cancer.

**When Julie was diagnosed with breast cancer, she was devastated and did not know what to do.** Her doctors advised her to take advantage of the conventional cancer treatments available to her. Standard cancer treatments include radiation, chemotherapy, and surgery. Many people are terribly afraid and will dutifully follow their physicians' advice and choose these standard of care therapies, without considering any alternatives.

Julie called her cousin, Gertie, in Germany to ask for her advice. She remembered that Gertie had overcome her own breast cancer by going to a European cancer clinic. Julie was surprised when Gertie explained that biological-medicine-based cancer treatments are commonly used to treat cancer in Europe. Gertie told Julie that she had been treated at the Paracelsus Cancer Clinic[21] in Switzerland. Gertie explained that new patients in European cancer clinics are first examined by a biological dentist in the dental section of their clinic. Gertie went on to emphasize that the very first priority in these European cancer treatment centers is to clean up infections in the mouth, using supplements, nutrients, and therapies that can help improve the balance of good bacteria to bad bacteria in the mouth. This is in sharp contrast to the U.S., where standard treatment of infections in the mouth, usually with antibiotics or gum surgery, often does not help and is often toxic and harmful.

**The goal of the biological dentist is to remove any ongoing sources of toxicity coming from the mouth.** Often the sources of toxicity are the direct result of dental procedures performed by conventional dentists doing exactly what they were taught to do in dental school. Julie decided to follow the example of the European biologically-based cancer treatment centers. First, she followed a strict protocol to clean up the infections in her gums. Then she found a good biological dentist who removed her root-canal teeth, replaced her mercury fillings with biocompatible fillings (determined by a blood test), and had her cavitations in her jawbones cleaned out.

Julie's breast tumor shrank and vanished within a few months. All her tests now showed that the cancer was completely gone. Julie was ecstatic to be rid of the cancer. She was glad that she had chosen to treat her cancer with alternative methods. Instead of having to go through the often severe side effects produced by the standard-of-care cancer treatments of radiation, chemotherapy, and surgery, Julie was now feeling better than she had ever felt in her entire life. She remains cancer-free ten years later.

## 3. MY DENTAL DECEPTION AND HEALING.

**Next, please listen to my story.** This is a story of deception by respected dentists whom I trusted and the harmful dental procedures that led to health problems down the road. Fortunately, a biological dentist was able to correct the major causes of my health problems in just two hours.

**Periodontal disease (infection in gum and bone) had accelerated and my teeth were loosening.** I had to have two teeth extracted in the last year and would lose two more very soon.

My dentist's prediction was dire. He reported to me that, "One by one, each of your teeth will loosen and have to be removed in the near future."

I asked him, "Why am I suddenly losing my teeth?"

His answer was, "I don't know."

**I was not happy with my dentist's dire outlook for my teeth.** I like having teeth to chew my food and don't relish the thought of getting dentures. But the way things were going, I sensed that his prediction for rapid tooth loss was probably right. His inability to tell me why I was losing my teeth was my cue to look for another dentist, one who understood the causes of tooth loss and would help me to stop this insidious progression.

It just didn't make sense. I am very careful with my diet. I avoid sugar, gluten, dairy, and processed food. I eat plenty of vegetables, fruits, and wild-caught salmon. I get plenty of exercise and I take good care of my teeth. I use bioidentical hormones, which keep my bones strong. (We discuss bioidentical hormones in several of our books.)[22] So I thought back through my dental history searching for the reason for the tooth loss that was occurring now in my sixties.

I began to review the research available about the consequences of common dental procedures. What I found was shocking.

I found that the dental procedures that had been done in my mouth over the course of my life were not only directly responsible for the tooth loss that I was now experiencing, but also contributed to the immune challenges (allergies, asthma, hypothyroidism, and poor digestion) that I now faced. For the past year, I had also felt serious pain behind my right eye, making it difficult to sleep. This pain could also be traced to dental and other traumas.

This revelation of the association between dental work and my current health woes was absolutely stunning, because I had trusted every dentist who worked in my mouth as an authority figure whom I assumed had my best interests at heart. Let's look back at my dental history and examine exactly what had happened to me.

## Improper extraction, scar tissue, and braces.

**As a young child, I had an extra tooth in the front of my upper jawbone (maxilla) removed.** My parents had no idea that the improper extraction techniques of this tooth would contribute to pain behind my eye much later on in life. Also contributing to the pain behind my eye much later in life was an eye operation to correct a lazy eye, performed when I was two. Breaking my nose a few times as life went on had added more scar tissue deep inside my head.

**My parents also paid more money than they could afford for braces on both upper and lower jaws.** The braces caused me to withdraw socially, as I perceived myself to be a hideous caricature of my real self. Even worse, the braces tore up the inside of my lips, causing painful swollen gashes. The braces also led to headaches. When a wire broke on the inside of my lower teeth, my orthodontist chastised me severely for allowing my tongue to go inside of the wire that he had misplaced. After several years of braces, I was glad to get them off and be rid of this tormenting dentist who tightened the braces up painfully every month and yelled at me to boot.

After the braces came off, I still had headaches caused by the loss of the natural movement of the bones in my head. Those headaches lasted for thirty more years, until I was treated by an osteopathically-trained physician, who helped restore the natural movement of the bones in my head.

## Massive mercury poisoning.

**I never had a cavity in my life until I went to college.** The dentist at U.C. Santa Barbara, where I attended college, shocked me when he informed me that I had 14 cavities.

I thought that it was odd that there was a sudden explosion of cavities in my mouth. I had received a dental check-up and cleaning every six months for my whole life and a cavity had never been spotted before.

**I blindly trusted this authority figure.** It did not occur to me that this dentist might be taking advantage of my dental insurance company.

**He drilled my teeth, and filled them with "silver" fillings.** He followed the philosophy of, "Drill 'em, fill 'em, and bill 'em." The more he could drill and fill, the more he could bill.

Immediately afterward, I became very ill, dizzy, and went deaf with a loud buzzing in my ears. Within a few months, I had regained my hearing.

**Then, just a year later, another dentist said all my fillings were badly done and replaced all of them again with more silver fillings.** After that I developed serious allergies and asthma, which did not go away. Twenty years later, it came to my attention that the silver fillings in my mouth contained the extremely toxic heavy metal, mercury, known to cause many diseases and serious health problems.

**I found a dentist who safely removed all of the toxic fillings that contained mercury and other heavy metals.** He replaced the fillings with white porcelain (composite) fillings. Although the composite filling material did contain tiny amounts of aluminum, it was a lot better than the hugely toxic mercury-laden fillings.

**This dentist told me to be quiet about the fact that he had removed the mercury fillings and replaced them with composites.** He said that other dentists had their licenses revoked for doing this, and he didn't want to get his license yanked. This was stunning, yet true.

The standard of care of dentistry that allows a highly toxic poison to be placed in a patient's mouth is very threatened by the vast research showing this to be a highly-negligent practice. Therefore, dentists who remove amalgams and do not replace them with more amalgams are subject to attack by their state's dental board.

**I began to realize that the dental profession was being regulated by authorities with ulterior motives that had nothing to do with health and a lot to do with big business.** I appreciated his candor and his courage to do what is right in spite of peer pressure to follow the status quo's culture of corruption.

**I got tested for heavy metals and found that I did have high levels of mercury, as well as other metals.** I began protocols to remove the toxic metals from my body. I knew that I was lucky to finally have this terrible mercury poison removed from my mouth and the rest of my body. I began to wonder why it was that the first two dentists used mercury in their fillings. And I wondered if there had never been any cavities in the first place. I never had any cavities before or after that dentist in Santa Barbara drilled, filled, and billed.

**It occurred to me that perhaps making money was more important to some dentists than having integrity.** Mercury has been proven to be highly toxic. In fact, it is one of the most toxic heavy metals that exist on this planet.

## Jawbone infection caused by dental procedures.

**Like many kids, I had to have my wisdom teeth pulled.** Having my wisdom teeth extracted was a truly miserable experience. The general anesthesia made me sick for a week. And the swelling in my jaws was super painful. What I didn't know was that this ordeal was going to be a time bomb, leading to the destruction of my jawbones from chronic infections in the bones at the extraction sites.

**The next tooth to go was one of my front upper incisors.** After a root canal procedure a few years before, the tooth finally had to be extracted, as the bone around it became more and more infected.

**A molar had also received a root canal treatment.** This resulted in more smoldering infection seeping into my maxilla (upper jaw) and, via the blood circulation, into my whole body. Without knowledge of what was happening and blindly trusting my dentists' wisdom in performing these procedures, my health had slowly deteriorated over the years.

**What I didn't realize when I got the root canal procedures and the extractions was the negative consequences of each of these dental procedures as time went on.** I later learned that root canal procedures leech toxic poisons into the body. I also learned that the way a dentist performs an extraction can lead to bone problems down the line.

True biological dentists understand this. They do not perform root canals, and they remove all teeth that have root canals. They also take precautions to prevent future problems in the bones around extraction sites. If a dentist calls himself a biological dentist, but still does root canals and uses improper extraction techniques, keep looking for a real biological dentist. We will give you a list of questions to ask a dentist to determine the facts about his or her procedures.

**After the extraction of the front tooth, the dentist wanted to implant a fake tooth into the roof of my mouth.** Implant surgery is very profitable. He made it seem like the only sane choice. He did not tell me about any harmful consequences of implants. The $7000 he wanted to charge me wasn't my only reason for not wanting to go along with his advice to get the implant. I already had knowledge about the negative consequences of implants, facts that he was not sharing with me.

**I knew that an implant could spell bad news for me.** As a bodyworker, I had once treated a patient who had suffered infections in the bones in her head as a result of a dental implant. After the dentist implanted an artificial tooth into her maxilla (roof of the mouth), she developed a massive infection with extreme headaches, and then developed severe health problems. I immediately sent her to see a dentist who removed the implant.

Unfortunately, we were too late. She never overcame the infection and resulting health problems. The headaches and ill health continued until she passed away a few years later.

**Another option my dentist presented to me was to get a bridge that would permanently connect an artificial tooth to the teeth on either side.** Again, I had knowledge of the negative consequences of this procedure as well, information that was not being presented to me by my dentist. The problem with the bridge option is that the bridge would cross the midline of my maxilla. The maxilla is the bone that forms the roof of the mouth. The maxilla has a suture (moving joint) that runs down the middle of it. A bridge would lock up that suture and prevent my head bones from expanding and contracting with the cranial-sacral rhythm.

**This bridge could cause headaches and more health problems all over the body.** This was definitely not a reasonable option from my viewpoint.

**So I opted to get a removable partial denture instead.** As it isn't very comfortable, I don't wear it much. It does restrict the motion of my head bones when I do wear it. The good news is that, unlike a permanent bridge, I can take it out. So I only wear it when I am going someplace where I feel that my appearance is important. As time goes on, I wear the partial less often. I am beginning to prefer to have the innocent look of a 7-year old with a front tooth missing. After all, who needs vanity? It is greatly over-rated. As an added bonus, it seems to me that people think I am more interesting without that front tooth and often open up to me more easily. Sure, some people are horrified. No big deal. Their shock is actually interesting to me. Not having a front tooth also reminds me to be more humble.

**As life went on, I lost more teeth.** None of these teeth were lost due to decay. Just like the front tooth, they had to go because of bone problems. As the bone around the two rear molars on the lower jaws (one on each side) dissolved, these molars just became loose and needed to be extracted. The question, "Why is this happening?" begged to be answered.

Soon thereafter, I needed to have two more molars extracted, this time from the upper jaw. One of the molars to be extracted was a perfectly fine tooth, except for the fact that the bone underneath it had been eaten away. The other molar had a gold crown and had undergone a root canal procedure. Pulling them out would not affect my ability to chew food, because neither molar had an opposable molar underneath, as those had been extracted last year.

**Before deciding on a dentist to pull these teeth, I set out to find out why my teeth were literally falling out of my jaws.** There had to be a reason for *why* my bones had decided not to hang on to my teeth anymore. I also had a sneaking suspicion that the nagging pain I was having behind my right eye when I tried to sleep had something to do with what was going on in my mouth.

**The answers to my questions were not easy to find.** I consulted several dentists, but they were not giving me any information. There wasn't anything on the internet either. So I dug deeper and I prayed for answers to my questions about the reasons for my jaw disintegration and my eye pain.

Suddenly I hit pay dirt! I spent the next few months listening to technical lectures given by experts in the field of biological dentistry. These experts often spoke in complicated medical terms. I was grateful that my medical background allowed me to understand what they were saying.

Unbeknownst to me, my lower jawbone (mandible) and upper jawbone (maxilla) were being eaten away by silent, smoldering infections deep within the bones. The technical term is osteonecrosis of the jawbones or cavitations. This was the real reason why my teeth were becoming loose and requiring extraction.

**I kept studying and learned exactly how to pull myself out of the dental trap into which I had fallen.** I began to understand that I needed to see a good biological dentist who would help me to reverse the problems in my mouth in order to improve my health and prevent future health problems.

## Going to the biological dentist.

Previous dental work had initiated a cascade of events that was slowly destroying my jawbones, destroying my immune system, causing terrible pain behind my right eye, and leading to ever-worsening chronic diseases. I had blindly trusted all of the other dentists who had worked in my mouth, thinking that they had been trained by a system that had my best interests at heart. I was wrong.

**This time, I had thoroughly done my homework.** After spending months researching biological dentists, I made plans to see an excellent biological dentist who had set up his practice in Tijuana, Mexico. I had gone to a local dentist to get 3D X-rays and then sent copies off to some of the best biological dentists in the world. Dr.

Lagos came out on top in my estimation. I knew that I could trust him. Dr. Lagos came highly recommended by Huggins Applied Healing.

**These dentists trained by Dr. Huggins began calling themselves "biological dentists."** Biological dentists consider the whole biology of the person being treated.

**Dr. Hal Huggins had trained Dr. Lagos in his system of total dental revision.** Dr. Huggins insisted upon removing all of the dental causes of ill health including amalgam fillings, root canals, and cavitations. This is what he meant by total dental revision. Conditions that may respond to total dental revisions include relief of chronic fatigue,[23] M.S.,[24] [25] brain fog, leukemia,[26] and cognitive problems.[27]

Dr. Huggins was a rebel who, when he discovered the serious flaws in the whole dental training system, was not afraid to publicly denounce established dental practices. Dr. Huggins criticized the practice of using toxic metals in dental materials. Dr. Huggins pronounced root canals to be vastly more toxic even than mercury fillings. And digging deeper, he found that standard extraction procedures were causing silent jawbone infections, called cavitations.

All of these flawed dental procedures had led to untold misery in the unwitting victims. Who were the victims? Well, most of us.

Of course, Dr. Huggins' outspoken criticism of flawed dental procedures did not win him favor with the Colorado Dental Board. They yanked his license. That did not stop him. Dr. Huggins was adamant that people receive proper dental treatment that did not harm their health. He began training a few select dentists in his work.

One of those dentists was Dr. Lagos. Dr. Lagos wanted me to send him a detailed lifetime health and dental history along with the 3D X-rays. I sent him a five page summary. He also asked me to see an oral surgeon to clarify a bubble seen on the 3D X-ray. The bubble was going into the sinus cavity from the tooth with the root canal.

After learning that it was not a concern, he agreed to see me in two months. I got our passports renewed and made all the travel arrangements.

**To make our way to Mexico, my husband and I jetted to San Diego.** As it was late, we caught a cab to a San Diego motel and overnighted. In the morning we grabbed breakfast and then hopped onto the trolley for a pleasant one-hour ride to the border. After a half hour wait, we cleared customs and grabbed a cab to get some food for our room and then went on to our very nice motel room in the Playas (beach) district of Tijuana. This part of Tijuana is relatively safe. Tijuana is now a lot cleaner than I remembered it from the last time I had been there twenty years ago. Everyone was very nice to us. We even received special treatment at a seafood restaurant, where we were ushered to a table without having to wait in line. The next morning we walked a few blocks over to Dr. Lagos' office. As I filled out the paperwork I was astonished to see something I had never seen before on the paperwork in a dentist's office.

**IT WAS AN INFORMED CONSENT FORM.** Most dentists don't tell you if they are going to do anything that might harm your health down the line. Not Dr. Lagos. Dr. Lagos is an honest man. He was stating his philosophy right here for you to agree with or walk. His philosophy mirrored that of Dr. Hal Huggins and the Huggins Applied Healing, where he was trained. I agreed with that philosophy and signed the consent form. I gave the previously agreed-upon cashiers' check to Adam, Dr. Lagos' secretary.

After a few minutes, Dr. Lagos told me to go to the bathroom and then led me into the immaculately clean operating room, where I made myself comfortable in the dental chair. I was introduced to Ricardo, the anesthesiologist, and Dr. Lagos' other assistants.

Dr. Lagos, standing at my side, spoke perfect English.

"We are monitoring your blood pressure. It is 135 over 80."

"A little high, but understandable," I said.

"Yes. We will be watching it throughout the whole procedure."

Then Ricardo began drawing blood. He needed a lot, because they were going to make platelet-rich plasma (PRP) with it.

**The PRP would be used to cover the surgical sites before stitching them up.** The PRP encourages fast healing. As I was having eight cavitations cleaned out, they would need a lot of blood. Ricardo was making noises that indicated he was not happy with the way this blood was being drawn out. There were some words in Spanish that I did not quite understand. My Spanish is pretty good, but I had not learned these particular phrases in my Spanish texts. I decided that Ricardo was probably a perfectionist. That is a good trait to have in an anesthesiologist. Dr. Lagos calmly explained that we were doing great, but we would have to open another vein to get more blood. No big deal.

**So we finally got all the blood drawn and we began the Vitamin C and the conscious sedation drip into that same vein.** The Vitamin C prevents infections and promotes fast healing. Conscious sedation is using medication to put you to sleep, but not so deeply asleep that you can't respond to requests if needed. With conscious sedation, if the dentist tells you to turn your head, you will do that. The only thing is, you don't remember a thing. I am going to vote conscious sedation two thumbs up. I was not groggy afterward and experienced no pain during and after the procedure.

I had previously had teeth extracted with standard dental anesthesia (injections of local anesthetic, like Novocain) and general anesthesia. I suffered during the procedures and for many days afterward with pain and grogginess. For extensive procedures like those I was facing, I will give standard dental anesthesia and general anesthesia two thumbs down.

Last thing I remembered was a tug on a molar that was being extracted. It actually felt pleasant. That was all I remembered until Dr. Lagos told me that they were done. I noticed something taped to my face.

**Dr. Lagos explained that the magnets on my face would also speed healing.** "Everything went perfect," he reassured me. Tears were running down my face from the right eye that had been plaguing me for over a year. Tears continued to flow for ten minutes. Then he led me to another room where he covered me with a blanket. I was a little shocky.

**A massage therapist came in and did a bit of cranial acupressure and then I fell asleep for about a half hour.**

Dr. Lagos came in and said to me, "I bet you don't remember that I said I had some money to give back to you."

"NO! I would have remembered that!" I exclaimed.

"Yes. I am going to give you back $850. We did not need as much anesthesiology as we had billed."

I was thinking, "Hallelujah! Our checking account was nearly tap city paying for this dental visit and the trip involved."

Not only did Dr. Lagos masterfully perform the work I needed to be able to overcome my chronic health problems, but he did it for a small fraction of the cost that the other dentists wanted to charge me. And now he is giving me money back? I must have died and gone to heaven!

That night I slept propped up on my back, so as not to disturb the blood clots. When we appeared at Dr. Lagos' office the next morning, the report was good. The clots were intact and I was healing nicely.

Dr. Lagos asked me if I had needed the pain pills he had given me. "Nope. I didn't have any pain."

"No pain at all?"

"Nope."

"What about discomfort?"

"Nothing. Seriously. My mouth has not hurt at all. I did stub my toe though and that hurts like crazy."

Dr. Lagos and his assistant, Alexandra, beamed at each other. And then Dr. Lagos gave me the $850, all in cash. Sweet.

We stayed another night, even though I felt well enough to go home that day. As I knew that chewing would be out of the question, I had requested a blender for our room. I discovered that I could blend a seafood soup and sip that.

The next day we cabbed to the border. When we got to the front of the line, the customs agent asked me, "What's that on your face?'

"Magnets."

"Why do you have magnets on your face?"

"Oral surgery. Helps the healing."

"Why do you have magnets? Do you have metal in your mouth?"

"Not anymore." I had a tooth with a gold crown removed, so this was now true.

"Then why the magnets?"

"These are very special magnets. You only get these from a very progressive dentist who knows how to speed healing tremendously. That's why I came to Tijuana."

"Oh, OK. I never saw that before. Go ahead."

My husband and I were very glad to hop that trolley back up to our motel in San Diego near the airport. We dropped our bags there and headed over to a special juice place we had found the first day. I ordered four large beet treats and drank them all down. I was starved.

The next morning we flew home. I was never so glad to see my Blend-tec. Everything I ate was blended until day five after the surgery. Then I began to eat soft foods. I applied ozonated olive oil to my gums to prevent infection and aid healing. For another month, I continued to wear the magnets, moving them around on my face.

There was quite a bit of aching in my right jaw joint that continued on and off for about six weeks. But overall, everything healed up quickly. The pain behind my right eye gradually began to resolve, hurting less and less every night. The scar tissue in my nose and face seemed to be dissolving, and I felt the pain moving around.

**Then about six weeks later, I awoke one morning with no pain at all behind my eye.** I was overjoyed. That is when I knew for sure that the treatment had really worked. My allergies and asthma also had subsided and my digestion had improved.

## Question everything.

**My experiences have taught me that we need to take responsibility for our own health, without blindly following the advice of trusted authorities.** Our conventional health-care system in the U.S. is symptom-based, ignoring the causes of ill health, and often makes health worse by using toxic drugs, radiation, and chemotherapy. Rather than calling it a health-care system, a more accurate description of this system would be to call it a disease-care system. Let's choose to be healthy for our whole life. To do that, you may need to question authority.

**If you want to protect yourself and your family from sickness, you must evaluate everything that goes into your body or touches your body.** To ensure that you are not taking in toxins, you have to get completely disciplined about everything.

**Never forget that you are in charge of your own health-care, even if you have found health-care providers who claim to be holistic.** Question everything. If your dentist wants to treat your symptoms without looking for the causes of your problems, it may be time for you to look for a dentist who seeks to discover the underlying causes of your health problems.

**Many dentists do not have the knowledge that is necessary to protect you from harm.** We have been led to believe that all health professionals know what is best for us when it comes to their specialty field, and that we should trust these authorities. But the truth is, you *can't* blindly trust a health professional to do what is in your best interests. The financial health of your dentist may come before your best interests.

**The philosophy followed by the majority of dentists in the U.S. maximizes profit by trying to save all of the teeth with the cheapest possible treatment**. They assume that long-term toxic effects of dental treatments are irrelevant or non-existent, and that all teeth should be saved at all costs. This leaves the toxic long-term consequences to the medical doctors.

**Is it worth it to save a tooth if the procedure leads to disease and death?** Is it worth it to save a tooth at the expense of damaging your immune system and your health? It's your call.

It helps if you understand this choice before you make a decision about getting a dental procedure. A conventional dentist will not tell you about the long-term negative consequences. Unlike medical doctors, dentists are not expected to obtain your informed consent.

**Read on to understand the long-term effects of the procedures commonly performed by conventional dentists.** This book will help you to understand exactly what options you really do have about your dentistry and your health. What exactly are the consequences of those common dental procedures your dentist is performing on you and your family? Is it possible that the most common dental procedures practiced by nearly all dentists put you at a high risk for life-threatening illness?

## 4. DISEASES CAUSED BY MOUTH PROBLEMS.

**Dental disease underlies more health problems than is commonly recognized.** Perhaps you think that you are doing fine and don't have any real health problems. But if you look more closely, there may be symptoms of ill health. Your symptoms may still be mild, such as fatigue, memory problems, depression, indigestion, or allergies. Even minor problems like memory issues, canker sores, poor digestion, and headaches have an underlying cause.

**Often the first symptom of ill health to appear is fatigue.** Fatigue is a common complaint that doctors hear from their patients. If you frequently feel tired, don't ignore this important red flag.

**What starts out as a small health problem may progress to other end of the health spectrum.** Problems in the mouth may cause much more serious diseases that may become life-threatening.[28] These include M.S. (multiple sclerosis),[29] lupus,[30] rheumatoid arthritis,[31] [32] A.L.S. (Lou Gehrig's disease),[33] Parkinson's,[34] Alzheimer's,[35] cardiovascular disease,[36] HIV,[37] diabetes,[38] low birth weight and pre-term birth,[39] osteoporosis,[40] brain aneurysms,[41] as well as many different forms of cancer.[42]

**The question we must ask ourselves if we want to recover our health is, "Why are we sick?"** We need to search for the causes and eliminate them. Many people find that health problems disappear when problems in the mouth are addressed.[43] Don't be surprised if heart arrhythmias disappear after having root-canal treated teeth extracted and mercury fillings removed and replaced with biocompatible fillings. It is not at all uncommon. Sinus problems may also clear up. Bloodwork may improve. Autoimmune problems, cancer, heart disease, and facial pain may become history. Diverse health problems of many kinds often disappear. Even back problems may go away.

**Physical issues in the mouth disturb the electrical signals that go to the rest of the body.** Chinese medicine considers the electrical meridians. Every meridian in the body goes to a tooth. If you have a dead tooth or a root canal on a first molar, the tooth cannot give out the energy that it should to the large intestine. The reverse is possible. If the organ has a problem, it may cause the tooth to hurt because the energy isn't coming back properly from the organ. Wisdom teeth are on the same meridian as the heart and low back. Rheumatological disorders, such as frozen shoulder, or soft tissue rheumatism may also be caused by a disruption in the signals along this meridian. Here is a link to an interactive dental meridian chart. http://www.mymercuryfreedentist.com/meridianChart.shtml You can see which organ shares electrical signals with each tooth. You can also see which emotion is tied to which tooth. Removing root canal teeth can improve mood, even improving debilitating cases of depression and other emotional problems. This can happen very soon after the removal of the dead root canal treated teeth.

## Cancer.

**The organ affected by cancer is often on the same meridian as a root canal tooth.** Using a thermal camera, a hot spot in the body may be found to be related to a hot spot in the mouth. Both hot spots can be seen on the same meridian. For instance, a tumor in the breast can be seen with the thermal camera. A hot spot may also be seen on the #2 tooth or on the #15 tooth, whichever is on the same side as the breast tumor. These teeth are on the breast meridians.

**A weak immune system cannot protect the body against the growth of cancer, and eventually succumbs to the disease.** Dr. Joseph Issels in Germany was a pioneer in treating cancer by addressing challenges to the immune system.[44] Dr. Issels said that 98% of his advanced cancer patients had between two and ten dead teeth.[45] [46] These dead teeth were often root canal treated teeth. Gum disease, cavitations in the jawbones, and root canals are all sources of infections that spread to the rest of the body. They all cause inflammation. The immune system becomes weakened from continually having to fight off infection.

The tonsils are often involved in seeding toxicity to other parts of the body,[47] especially if the person has or has ever had a root canal. The tonsils become overwhelmed with the huge amount of toxicity coming from the root canal. Even if the tonsils look OK, they may still be infected. The infection may only become evident when they are removed. Dr. Issels got good results in treating metastatic cancer when he included tonsil removal along with root-canal teeth removal as part of his protocol. If your blood tests still show infection, and you have done everything else to remove it, (cleaned out your mouth, cleaned up your digestion) you may want to seriously consider having your tonsils removed.[48]

## Autoimmune disease.

**The incidence of autoimmune disease is exploding.** Twenty million Americans have autoimmune disease.[49] Most people with autoimmunity don't know that they have it. They have not even recognized that their health problems are a form of autoimmunity.[50] Women are 60% more likely to have autoimmune disease than men.[51]

In autoimmunity, the immune system sends out antibodies and attack cells that attack different parts of the body. In an autoimmune state, the immune system can no longer tell the difference between the good guys and the bad guys. It misidentifies your own tissues as a foreign invader. The immune system attacks the joints (arthritis), nose (allergies), thyroid, or just about any other place you can think of.

**Autoimmunity can be reversed.** Infections in the mouth may play a big part in causing this over-activity of the immune system. Elevated antibodies must be lowered by decreasing inflammation in the body, especially the mouth. When someone has autoimmune disease, the first thing that must be done is to work on getting rid of the worst causes of inflammation. Then systematically work on removing each of the other causes in order of severity. Amy Meyers, M.D. in her book, "The Autoimmune Solution," discusses five causes of autoimmunity that must be addressed if the disease is to be overcome.[52]

- **Infections.** Bacterial infections, fungal infections, and viruses (Epstein Barr virus, herpes virus, and other viruses) all contribute to autoimmunity.[53] Root canals, gum disease, and jawbone disease are a source of silent bacterial infections.[54] Consulting a biological dentist is important to remove mercury fillings, root canals, and overcome bone infections.
- **Diet issues.** The biggest problems are with processed food filled with herbicides, pesticides, GMO's, sugar, caffeine, preservatives, and chemicals.[55] Dr. Meyers recommends that people with autoimmune conditions remove all processed food, grains, dairy, eggs, legumes, seeds, nuts, and nightshades from the diet. I have found that her dietary recommendations are the strictest of all of the health gurus, but they are also the most effective, because they remove all of the dietary triggers of autoimmunity.
- **Intestinal permeability (leaky gut).** This is most often caused by food sensitivities to the gluten found in grains, and problems digesting legumes, dairy products, eggs, nuts, and seeds. Eliminate these foods to heal leaky gut.
- **Environmental toxins.** We are exposed to over 80,000 in our environment. They build up in your body as time goes on if you don't cleanse them out. Mercury fillings are a major cause of heavy metal toxicity.[56][57]
- **Stress.**[58] Modern life is full of low-level and not-so-low-level stresses. The stress hormones suppress the immune system.

## Cardiovascular disease.

**Toxicity in our mouths may be the underlying cause of heart problems.**[59] The latest studies are showing that heart disease is caused by an inflammatory process. Dental infections cause inflammation that feeds heart disease. In the vast majority of cases of people who have bacteria in the blood, the pathogens are being seeded by disease in the mouth. These are very potent toxins, more toxic than Botulism.[60] With every bite, toxins are draining from the teeth into the bloodstream. Chewing generates enormous pressures on the drainage of the veins from the mouth. Root canals are most often done on the molars, where the chewing forces are greatest. The more advanced the cardiovascular disease, the more periodontal and root canal pathogens are found in the plaque of the blood vessels.[61]

**The bacteria that cause gum disease are found in the arteries of people with heart disease.**[62] [63] Gum disease significantly increases risk for stroke.[64] The bottom line is that in many heart patients the infections in root canals, infected gums, and tonsils are the underlying causes of their heart disease.[65] It is critical to address the problems in the mouth if these patients are to overcome their cardiovascular disease.

**The root-canal tooth is chronically infected, even if the pain goes away.** The bacteria travel from the mouth to the heart to the plaque in the coronary arteries, rupturing the plaque and causing heart disease.[66] [67] Chronically infected tonsils or a constipated gut with infectious disease can also cause pathogens to seed into the arteries and veins.

## Facial pain.

**Facial twitches may be the result of heavy metal poisoning.** Mercury from dental fillings is a likely suspect in facial twitches. The solution is to see a biological dentist who will safely remove amalgam fillings and then begin a detoxification program to remove mercury from your body.

**Sometimes an area of poorly healed jawbone may harbor low grade infection that can impact your overall health.** If a nerve becomes impacted by a cavitation, it may cause jaw pain, facial pain, and the very painful facial pain of trigeminal neuralgia.[68] Read the chapter on jawbone disease to discover exactly how disease in the jawbone begins and progresses and what you can do to stop the disease and recover from facial pain.

## 5. CHOOSE YOUR DENTIST WISELY!

**If you go to a dentist who understands how to correct dental problems safely, you may be able to significantly improve your health.** On the other hand, if you go to a conventional dentist, especially one who performs root canals and uses mercury fillings and chemical mouthwashes, you may actually make yourself sicker.

People often blindly follow the advice of conventional dentists, not understanding how dangerous these therapies really are. Most people have no idea how seriously their health can deteriorate when they use the services of conventional dentists. Conventional dentistry can contribute to your health problems by increasing your body's toxic burden of metals and chemicals. Neurological[69] and autoimmune[70] effects follow exposure to mercury and other heavy metals. Other dental problems that lead to disease include jawbone cavitations and root canal treated teeth. The problem is, most dentists are not aware of the research and they have not been trained to be aware of these dental-treatment-caused health problems. We have had many advances in dentistry that have not been embraced by many dentists.

Many dentists have their primary focus on making people look good, but are doing so at the expense of their health. They could still make people look good without harming their health, if only they used non-toxic restorative materials. We have been led to believe that chemical mouthwashes are safe, but in reality, they are dangerous, especially for someone who has just had oral surgery. When the gums are bleeding, the chemicals are even more easily absorbed into the bloodstream.

### Conventional dentists use toxic treatments.

**Going to a conventional dentist is like going to a conventional doctor.** Just as you can get mercury fillings removed by a conventional dentist, your conventional doctor knows how to run some kinds of tests. But neither of these conventional health-care professionals may know how to do these procedures safely or properly.

**Health professionals can only be as good as the training that they have received.** If they wanted to graduate and get that degree, they had to agree with what was being taught in their medical or dental school. Most never questioned the safety and long-term repercussions of the treatments that they learned to perform in their training.

**Many dentists have faulty belief systems.**
- Many dentists believe that mercury is not harmful, despite massive evidence showing mercury's toxicity. If they do not believe that mercury is harmful, they will not take precautions to protect you, themselves, and the environment when handling mercury.
- Their belief that root canals are warranted and safe is another faulty belief system that has jeopardized the health of millions.
- A dangerous faulty belief held by most conventional dentists is that the procedures done in the mouth have nothing to do with the health of your other body tissues.

They may become upset if you challenge their beliefs. Don't be surprised if you find that a health professional becomes uncomfortable if you start asking questions about the potential problems that might result from their treatment methods. This means that you are questioning their authority and their belief systems. That belief system is being forced upon dentists by institutions that may punish them when they remove an amalgam for health reasons, rather than obvious dental problems. Dental schools still perpetuate the use of amalgams today, even though the evidence against using mercury is strong. If prospective dentists were to first educate themselves in toxicology, they would not accept the belief system of using toxic treatments.

**Don't be afraid to trust your own intuition.** Your dentist or doctor does not always know what is best for you. Don't be afraid to get a second opinion or change dentists or doctors.

## Mercury-free is not good enough.

**Some dentists remove mercury fillings for purely cosmetic reasons.** Amalgams are ugly. But just because they will remove the amalgams doesn't mean that they know how to do it safely. In fact, dental schools do not routinely teach safe amalgam removal. These cosmetic dentists may cause you to become seriously poisoned with mercury by removing the ugly mercury amalgams without using safe protocols. This is why the dentist that you choose should not be just a mercury-free dentist. He or she should also be holistic or a biological dentist.

## A new breed of dentists challenges old methods.

**A new breed of dentists is challenging the use of the traditional dental procedures that are taught in dental schools.** These new, forward-thinking dentists are not afraid of going against conventional methods of dentistry. The new dentists see the connections between health in the mouth and health of the body. These new dentists understand that everything in the body is somehow connected to everything else. They understand that having a healthy mouth is critical to having a healthy body. If you have problems in your mouth, you will have problems in other parts of your body as well.

**The Hippocratic Oath tells medical practitioners to, "First, do no harm."** The new dentists hold themselves responsible to uphold this highest standard of treatment. Plenty of research proves that many of the old dental practices that are still being used today by the majority of dentists are not just harmful, but downright deadly. The new dentists have a high degree of moral integrity, refusing to practice any harmful dental procedures learned in dental school.

**The new dentists have learned how to treat dental problems without creating more problems.** Rejecting the methods they were taught to use in dental school, these dental pioneers embrace the latest technological breakthroughs in diagnostic instrumentation, laboratory analysis, and state-of-the-art dental materials. These new dentists eagerly stand by to help you heal the problems in your mouth.

Many of these problems were caused by dentists who were using toxic dental materials, placing root canals, and improperly extracting teeth. The old dentists used deadly treatments such as mercury (silver) amalgam fillings, root canals (always a bad idea), and extraction techniques that resulted in silent, yet festering cavitations (holes in the bones). Although the old dentists do not acknowledge the dangers involved in these common dental procedures, research shows that these treatments result in all manner of disease and may even cause death.[71][72][73][74]

**Sometimes old dentists see the light and become new dentists.** This happens when a dentist is not afraid to set aside a belief system that was ingrained in dental school, look at the evidence, and admit that there may be a better way to do things. This may require some soul searching. The dentist must be ready to forgive himself or herself for any harm that was caused by using techniques that he or she thought were best at the time that they were used.

### Shifting belief systems.

**Because of a shift in consumer demand for cleaner foods and cleaner dentistry, more and more dentists are making the shift to clean up their practice.** Dentists who continue to use mercury and fluoride are beginning to lose patients, as more and more people want to clean up the toxicity in their bodies. As consumers, we have the power to demand cleaner and less toxic dental practices.

**The practice of medicine and dentistry in the U.S. is dictated by the profits of the pharmaceutical companies.** They profit from sickness. Deadly products are given the seal of approval by the F.D.A. Just as thalidomide was F.D.A. approved before causing tremendous amounts of birth defects, so is mercury approved for dental fillings. For-profit industries compromise our health in pursuit of their own interests.

**In other countries, mercury has been banned in dentistry.** But in the U.S., mercury use in fillings is accepted as safe and is still being taught in dental schools. We have warnings about mercury contamination in tuna. But it is still OK to put mercury into our mouths in the form of dental fillings.

**When dentists poison people with mercury and other toxins like fluoride, they are contributing to the suffering of many people.** Dentists who have been using toxic procedures for many years resist change, because they do not want to admit that what they have been doing has been causing harm.

When research proves that there is a better way to do something, as a rule, it takes about 18 years until the better method is taught in schools. If we want to progress more quickly, it is up to us, as consumers, to be open-minded and educate ourselves about the advances that are being made to heal ourselves from disease using the latest research discoveries.

**Look for a dentist who is not afraid to look at you as a "whole" interconnected human being.** Find a dentist who understands the toxicity of these substances and will respect your health. You choose where to spend your health-care dollars. When you seek help from a health-care practitioner of any kind, look at their own health and their attitude toward you and your questions. You are in charge of building a better team around you.

The idea of "holistic" is that the dentist looks at the body as a whole. But any dentist can call themselves holistic. They can even join holistic organizations without any training. A fee is all that is required to get their name on a list on the internet. You need to find out where they were trained, what procedures they use, and most importantly, talk to some of their patients. Talk to other people who are health-minded and find out what dentists they use.

## Biological dentists perform a total dental revision.
**Biological dentists prioritize cleaning up the mouth:**
- Close attention is paid to restoring good bacteria and overcoming the bad bacteria.
- Silent, smoldering infections are treated with natural remedies, instead of chemical poisons and antibiotics.
- Mercury fillings and root canal teeth are immediately removed.
- Cavitations, or holes in the jawbone, caused by improper extractions and infections, are opened up and thoroughly cleaned out.

**Biological dentists understand that if the mouth is not healthy, the body can't be healthy.** Biological dentists want to make sure that everything they do contributes to the health of the patient and that they do nothing which leads to illness. They understand that disease is caused by an overload of toxicity and not enough resources to get rid of it.

**A true biological dentist will perform a total dental revision to remove *all* of the dental causes of disease.** They understand that the toxins and materials used in the mouth can have harmful effects on overall health and only use materials that have been proven to be compatible to the immune system of the patient. They perform procedures that reverse the health problems caused by the actions of previous dentists.

Just like those calling themselves holistic dentists, any dentist can pay a fee and join organizations of biological dentists in order to get their name listed on that biological dentistry association's website. Some dentists who call themselves biological dentists may safely remove amalgam fillings, but they may also be doing root canals and implants. Only a very few will clean out cavitations. They may use materials that are not biocompatible to the patient's immune system.

The first thing that a good biological dentist will do is look inside the mouth for any causes of immune system aggravations. How many toxic heavy metal fillings, crowns, bridges, and implants are there? How many root canals and cavitations are there?

- Biological dentists take every possible precaution to avoid contamination when removing metal fillings.
- Biological dentists remove root canal teeth, toxic fillings, crowns, and implants.
- Biological dentists create new fillings, crowns, bridges, partials, and dentures made with materials that are biocompatible to the patient.
- Biological dentists clean out cavitations in the jawbones.

- Biological dentists do not do anything that will lead to disease in the future. Biological dentists do not put in implants or do root canal procedures.

**They are conservative in their use of antibiotics, using them only when absolutely necessary to kill off an infection.** They understand that a healthy microbiome of the mouth and gut is critical in preserving health.[75] Antibiotics kill off the good bugs as well as the bad bugs. Antibiotics, especially repeated rounds, decrease the diversity of bacteria in the microbiome. Many diverse kinds of bacteria in our mouths and guts ensure that our immune system remains healthy to protect us from disease.[76]

**Biological dentists also use state-of-the-art treatment modalities** to increase healing time, decrease pain, and increase the effectiveness of their treatments. These treatment modalities include high dose intravenous Vitamin C, conscious sedation, platelet rich plasma injections, acupressure, and magnets.

**Don't just assume that your dentist knows how to safeguard your health.** *You* must take matters into your own hands. Take an active role in improving your health. If you want to live a life free of chronic illness, it is important to thoroughly research the backgrounds of any health-care provider before entrusting your health to them.

**A good dentist's goal is to be of service to you.** Doctors who are willing to answer your questions are the ones you want to consider. Even if they can't do what you are looking for, there is a good chance that they may be able to refer you to someone who can.

**Ask the right questions.** Find out what protocols different dentists are using. When these dental procedures are performed correctly by a knowledgeable dentist, it can make a tremendous positive impact on your health. It is your right to find out how a prospective dentist feels about root canals. Ask them what they know about mercury toxicity.

**Educate yourself.** Read this book and implement the suggestions. A good dentist will encourage you to learn all that you can and to have an open mind about what is causing your health problems. Don't passively do whatever is recommended. If the dentist or doctor that you are consulting doesn't have the same philosophy of health care that you have, it will be impossible for you to get the results that you are seeking.

**Just because a dentist says that he or she can remove your amalgams safely, does not mean that they know how to do it safely.** Even if they are using a rubber dam in your mouth to keep you from swallowing mercury, this is not enough to ensure that the procedure is safe. Even if they have years and years of experience, this does not mean that they know how to do the procedure safely. A good dentist will use language that encourages the patient to accelerate their healing. A bad dentist uses fear to get the patient to accept toxic treatments. You have the choice to accept or reject any medical or dental intervention. It is your choice of who to go to. If you don't agree with the job the dentist is doing, you can go elsewhere. Find a dentist who will listen to you and uses holistic dentistry. Your goal is to find a dentist who will safely remove all the metal from your mouth and who will remove all infected teeth and properly diagnose and expertly clean your cavitations. After this is done, note improvements in your health. If symptoms return, you may still have another hidden infection, so go back to your dentist or find a better one who will properly diagnose all infections, even "silent" infections deep in the jawbone.

### Questions to ask a dentist. [77]

- What is your position on the mercury issue? The correct answer is that he or she is against the use of mercury in the mouth.
- Do you use a rubber dam when removing amalgam? The correct answer is yes, to prevent mercury particles from going down your throat.
- Do you utilize alternative air sources and/or equipment to reduce mercury inhalation? Is your suction system powerful and efficient? The correct answers are yes and yes. Mercury vapor must be removed from the office.
- Do you apply copious amounts of water to the filling upon removal? Correct answer is yes.
- Do you do root canals? Many dentists who call themselves biological dentists do root canals. Any dentist who would do a root canal is introducing a potent source of infection into your mouth. Step away from this dentist.
- Do you diagnose and treat cavitations? This one question alone will narrow your search considerably, as very few dentists are prepared to diagnose and properly treat cavitations.
- When you extract a tooth, do you remove the periodontal ligament and completely sterilize the area? The correct answer is yes, to prevent cavitations.
- Do you use epinephrine when doing extractions? The correct answer is no. Epinephrine prevents copious bleeding, which you want to prevent dry socket and cavitations.

## 6. DENTAL TOXINS.

**Of course, no ethical dentist would knowingly place a toxic material in a patient's mouth.** Those dentists who do place toxic dental materials into a person's mouth are usually unaware of the danger. Very few dentists are ever taught that patients can have a reaction to dental work. Those who do understand the dangers of certain dental materials may believe that only certain types of materials are reactive, and that by avoiding them, they can avoid any problems. This is not true.

**Anyone can have an immune reaction to any material, but some materials are more prone to causing an immune reaction than others.** Dental materials implanted into the teeth and jawbones expose the whole body to toxicity, creating the possibility of an immune response. Even composite or "porcelain" fillings usually contain aluminum. The aluminum shows up as bright and shiny on X-rays. To find out which materials you may react to, you have to get a biocompatibility test. It is advised to do this test before you have materials put into your mouth.

**Dental materials that people may react to include:**
- Mercury
- Cadmium.
- Copper.
- Zinc.
- Beryllium.
- Phenol.
- Aluminum.
- Nickel allergy is quite common and should not be used. It is sneaky, because the same nickel alloy that would make one's skin break out if used in an earring will not cause a rash in the mouth. Nickel in the mouth raises immune reactivity in the body. Stainless steel crowns are very toxic, especially those made of nickel and chromium.

## Mercury fillings expose you to a deadly poison.

**An amalgam ("silver") filling is a mixture of several metals, one of which is mercury.** Nickel, lead, aluminum, and cadmium are other problematic metals that are used in fillings. These metals do not stay in those fillings. They leech out of the fillings and are absorbed into the tissues of the body.[78] "Silver" fillings are made up of 50% mercury, which leeches out into the body, causing health problems.[79] This is the biggest source of mercury exposure for people who have them. Mercury fillings represent the largest mercury exposure to people all over the world. Dr. Friberg, the chief advisor of the World Health Organization, insists that there is no safe level of exposure to mercury.[80] [81]

**Mercury is one of the most toxic naturally-occurring substances in the world.**[82] Medical professionals realize this. In fact, if a mercury thermometer was still being used in a hospital and it broke, the whole floor would be closed down, and the haz-mat team would come in to clean it up. The dental filling has about fifty times as much mercury as a thermometer.

**Mercury exposure is deadly, affecting the way you think and feel.**[83] [84] If you have a mouth that contains one or more fillings that are made with mercury (amalgam or silver) fillings, you are constantly being exposed to toxicity.[85] When you chew or brush your teeth, mercury is released from the fillings and goes into your body's tissues. This happens from the very first day the mercury filling is placed into your mouth by a dentist, until it is removed. There is no safe way to place an amalgam filling.

Mercury amalgam is the absolute worst material being used to fill cavities. Careful barrier techniques are crucial when removing mercury to protect patient, doctor, and staff from mercury exposure during the procedure. Because the fillings do not last, they must be replaced repeatedly. But safety in removing mercury amalgams is usually not a priority in most dental offices. This causes toxic exposure not only to the patient, but also the dentist, dental personnel, and anyone in the office. The media is unaware of this problem. .

**Mercury vapor is released from amalgams**[86] **when you chew**[87] **and crosses right through the blood-brain barrier.** The more mercury you have in your mouth, the more mercury you have in your brain[88] and kidneys.[89] [90] It may take some time for symptoms to present themselves, as the mercury slowly builds up in the body. Early symptoms like fatigue, difficulty sleeping, anxiety, and depression may not be easily recognized as being associated with the amalgam fillings. Mercury from fillings can create many common symptoms including depression, anxiety, chronic fatigue,[91] chronic headaches, digestive upsets, depression, and memory problems.[92] Mercury toxicity in a pregnant woman and also in the father[93] can cause problems in the unborn child.[94] [95]

**Mercury causes destruction of your cells**[96] **and leaky membranes.**[97] Mercury vapor causes damage to both sciatic and optic nerves,[98] and nasal sinuses. Breathing in the mercury vapor takes the mercury straight into the brain,[99] damaging the lungs.[100] [101]

**Amalgams are a huge source of environmental pollution.**[102] The dental industry dumps about 4.4 tons of mercury into the planet every year. Mercury doesn't just come from coal-fired energy plants. It comes from dentists who keep putting it into people's mouths. Imagine the huge amount of mercury that is released into the environment when someone who has mercury fillings dies and is cremated.[103]

**In most dental offices, there are no procedures in place to remove the mercury from the air and the water.**[104] In both the U.S. and Canada, dental offices are the greatest polluters of ground water with mercury, when compared to all other industries. Dental assistants may be responsible for cleaning out the traps in sinks where mercury has collected. They often just flush these wastes down the toilet, where it is further distributed into our environment.[105]

In most dental offices, the problems with mercury have not been brought to their attention, or if they are aware of the problem, they have not taken steps to deal with mercury responsibly. When industrial EPA-type mercury "sniffers" (machines that detect mercury in the air) are brought into most dental offices, they typically record very high amounts of mercury in the air.[106] The International Academy of Oral Medicine and Toxicology (IAOMT) has discovered that the mercury vapor in most dental offices is so high, that if OSHA were to come in and find such high levels in any other business, they would shut them down.

Besides just the mercury vapor, another problem is particulate matter from the mercury being used in dental fillings. Particles of mercury are actually dropping onto the clothing and skin of the patients and dental professionals.

The mercury and other metals that are being used in dental offices often cause neurological problems in the personnel who work there,[107] because they are exposed to so much mercury in their environment.[108] Dentistry has a higher rate of mental illness than any other profession.[109] This statistic is caused by the use of mercury. Mercury is directly related to the development of sensory neuropathy. This is loss of feeling in the arms and legs.[110]

**Many people believe that the high rates of autism are caused by high heavy metal burdens, including mercury toxicity.** The mercury used in vaccines has been frequently blamed for autism. Some children with autism have been cured of the disease when they have undergone heavy metal chelation to remove the metals from their bodies.

If a mother has amalgams, eats farmed fish, and has had mercury-containing vaccinations, her mercury levels will be very high.

Studies are showing that the last generation has mercury levels 50% higher than the generation before. If the mother has high levels of mercury in her body, the offspring, especially the first, and especially if a boy, gets a huge dose of mercury. If the child is a boy, higher levels of testosterone dampen the detoxification pathways more than in a girl. Also, the first offspring generally takes on more heavy metals from the mother than later children. Very toxic mothers may have other autistic children, as well. When pregnant women get flu shots, they may not be aware that the manufacturers admit that the shots have not been tested on pregnant women, and that these flu shots bypass the immune system, and are going right into your tissues.

**Vaccines may damage children in several ways.** Even if they don't contain mercury, they may contain other toxic substances, like aluminum.[111] Particular care must be taken not to give them to a child who is very young, giving them too often, or to a sick child. Multi-dose vials are preserved with thimerosal, containing mercury.

**Mercury is especially toxic to the thyroid.** Many of us are deficient in iodine because our soils and foods are often very low in iodine. Mercury latches onto the thyroid molecule where the missing iodine belongs, rendering the thyroid molecule ineffective to do its job of keeping you feeling energetic and healthy.[112] [113] [114] When thyroid function is low, dental decay may be encouraged.[115]

**It is your responsibility to educate yourself, your family, and future generations about the dangers of mercury toxicity.** There are a few dental schools that are beginning to address the problems caused by mercury toxicity. It is important to find a dentist who has been properly trained, who follows a strict protocol, and who really respects your health by protecting you, protecting themselves, and protecting everyone in the office and in the world from mercury pollution.

### Five kinds of reactions to mercury.

**People react differently to mercury poisoning.**[116] Mercury always attacks the weakest system first. Some people have so many symptoms from mercury toxicity that doctors are baffled and prescribe anti-depressants, because they don't suspect that mercury toxicity is the cause and think that depression is the cause.

**There are five categories of reactions to mercury toxicity.**

(1) **Neurological** problems[117] can be sensory or motor. Sensory problems include brain fog, short-term memory problems, nervousness, and depression. Motor problems include tremors, leg cramps, and facial twitches.

(2) **Cardiovascular** problems include high blood pressure,[118] chest pains and tachycardia.[119]

(3) **Collagen** problems include joint pain and arthritis.[120]

(4) **Immunological** problems include autoimmune diseases,[121] when the body attacks its own tissues. Examples of autoimmune diseases caused by mercury poisoning are allergies, asthma, MS,[122][123] ALS,[124] lupus,[125] and some types of arthritis.[126] Mercury is so predictable in causing autoimmunity that it is used in animal studies to trigger the autoimmune disease that they wish to research.[127] Which autoimmune disease a person will develop is a factor of which genetic predisposition a person has.[128]

(5) **Miscellaneous** symptoms include ringing in the ears, hearing loss,[129] frequent urination, chronic fatigue, bloating after eating, metallic taste in the mouth, and hypothyroidism.[130] Chronic fatigue is due at least in part to insufficient oxygen availability. Red blood cells are particularly sensitive to toxic metals and anaerobic bacterial toxins.[131] Anaerobic bacteria are the nasty bacteria that live inside your gums and jawbones. The word anaerobic means that they live without air. Anaerobic bacteria produce toxic waste products that cause disease all over the body.[132][133][134] They have even been implicated in breast cancer.[135]

## Huggins protocol for amalgam removal.

**Safe removal of dental amalgams is a top priority.** Dr. Hal Huggins developed a safe protocol for the removal of mercury fillings. For greatest safety, they should be removed in a certain order. Dentists need to study with Huggins Applied Healing to learn how to do this. Huggins claimed that following his protocol leads to healing.[136]

To learn more about this protocol and to find a dentist who has been certified in Huggins' methodology, go to http://hugginsappliedhealing.com or call 1-866-948-4638, or E-mail: kim@drhuggins.com.

## Work with a holistic physician.

**When having mercury fillings and root canal teeth removed, it is good to simultaneously work with a holistic physician to provide support for the detox.** I.V. vitamin C is helpful to do before, at the same time, and after the dental revision procedure. Vitamin C helps you to remove the toxins and strengthens the immune system.

## Replacing fillings.

So what do you use to replace the amalgams after they are removed? Frequently dentists place a white filling that they call porcelain. It is not really porcelain. The term porcelain is used only because the filling is tooth colored. These white fillings are more accurately called composites. They are composed of a mixture of different materials. Composites may contain chemicals that may leach out--aluminum, acrylate, formaldehyde, hexane, hydroquinone, phenol, polyurethane, strontium, toluene, and xylene. Aluminum makes the composite filling last longer. Some composites can last as long as amalgam, but most of the time amalgam will outlive composites. The life of the filling is not that important. More important is how the dental fillings affect the life of the patient. The best question to ask when considering choice of dental fillings is, "Which materials are compatible to my body?" This is why it is important to get a compatibility test.

### Dental material compatibility testing.

**There are blood tests that can tell you which materials are more compatible with your immune system.**[137] The best materials to use are those that your body likes. It is sort of like getting a blood transfusion. You don't want to get Type B blood transfused if you are Type A. Biocompatibility tests measure the body's reactions to all of the different dental materials. Serum compatibility testing tells you which specific filling materials are best suited for each individual person. To get tested, you order a test kit, and then have your blood drawn and sent to a lab where they do Serum Biocompatibility Testing.

### Do you need bio-compatibility testing?

**People who are not particularly chemically sensitive may not need to be very concerned with compatibility testing for basic dentistry.** The newer, tooth-colored composite fillings and other non-metallic materials have caused fewer problems than the older metallic materials. We all have to put up with a bit of toxicity, immune reactivity, and galvanic stress.

**The more sensitive or the more unwell the person is, the more important it is to get the testing done.** Some people can't stand even minor stresses caused by common dental materials. These people usually know that they are the sensitive ones. If this is you, you need to get tested and insist upon biocompatible dental materials.

**Your dentist will tell you which lab to use. The two labs are:**
1. Clifford Consulting Laboratory, www.ccrlab.com, 719-550-0008
   Clifford grades products as either "satisfactory" or "unsatisfactory."
2. Biocomp Laboratories, www.biocomplabs.com, 800-331-2303
   Biocomp grades products as "highly reactive," "moderately reactive," and "least reactive."

Biocomp treats all aluminum the same, as a problem. Therefore they reject most porcelains and ceramics when aluminum sensitivity is detected.

Many more brands with aluminum end up on the good list in Clifford reports. Clifford labs says in their brochure that the form the aluminum takes is important, and that they will flag materials that contain aluminum that is not suited to a patient showing aluminum sensitivity.[138] Clifford regards insoluble aluminum compounds such as aluminum oxide and aluminum silicate as not biologically available, so products that contain aluminum in those forms are not graded "unsatisfactory" even if aluminum antibodies are detected.

### How to get tested.

**After your dentist tells you which lab to use, call the lab and have a test kit sent to you.** Your dentist will provide you with a prescription for a blood draw. Take the kit to a nearby blood lab, such as Quest Diagnostics, Labcor, or a local hospital. Fill out the enclosed paperwork and include payment. The blood lab draws one tube of blood, prepares frozen serum, and overnights the sample to the compatibility lab. It's best to draw the sample early in the week, so Biocomp or Clifford can receive it before the weekend. Both labs will get the results back to you quickly.

When your dentist receives the lab results, he or she can provide you with a list of acceptable materials from a Biocomp or Clifford test that he or she might consider using. The dentist might even give you a sample of the proposed material to take home and try out. You can hold it in your cheek for a few minutes or a few hours and see if a familiar reaction starts. Or you might want to try muscle testing or electrodermal testing to see if this material will work for you.

### Toxic crowns and bridges.

**It isn't just your fillings that are causing heavy metal toxicity in your body.** Crowns may also contain toxic metals. The most common crowns have cheap metals like nickel. Even the "gold" crowns have toxic metals like copper, silver, and palladium. Bridges may contain toxic materials also.

## Problems with metals in the mouth.

**Metal alloys cause electric currents in the mouth that often underlie health problems.** Oral galvanism has been talked about for well over 100 years, but dentists generally ignore it and its implications. When gold and titanium are grouped together in an electrolyte (like saliva), they have the potential to create a battery of over three volts. Every cell in your body is a little battery. Foreign energies, like galvanic responses and EMF's from your cell phone adversely affect the health of your energetic and physical body. This can commonly cause jaw tension, TMJ, temporal headache, and other problems.

### *Metal testing labs.*

**Sometimes we need to use metals in dentistry.** But before doing so, it may be important to test for sensitivity. Some metals, most notoriously nickel, will create contact dermatitis, or a skin rash, upon exposure, and these are easily discovered by history and by serum testing. Other metals, most notoriously titanium, will never make a skin rash, but can lead to weakness and other vague and varied symptoms. The most revealing metal sensitivity test is the Melisa (memory lymphocyte activation) test (www.melisa.org). This is the only test that will show titanium sensitivity.

## Fluoride is a toxic poison.

**Fluoride is another poison that dentists put in our mouths that hurts our health.**[139] Not only that, but many cities put it in our water. Studies show that cancer deaths increase when fluoride is added to the water.[140] [141] Fluoride is harmful to the bones,[142] connective tissue,[143] and the brain and nervous system.[144]

Fluoride is a toxic waste product that phosphate fertilizer companies are happy to pawn off on toothpaste manufacturers and public water suppliers. The more it is used, the greater the damage to the central nervous system.[145] It should never be used in dentistry or in any product. Putting it in drinking water is criminal. It is not helpful at all. It does not prevent tooth decay. It causes dental problems over time. Excess fluoride accumulation in the teeth causes fluorosis, or damage to the tooth structure.

Treating our children's teeth with fluoride rinses and varnishes is a potent source of fluoride poisoning. The children swallow it.

**Evidence shows that continual fluoride exposure leads to the dumbing down of our kids.**[146] We know that fluoride harms their neurological development. Fluoride has been found to lower children's I.Q.[147] [148] [149] [150] [151] The use of fluoride is a crime against our children.

**Fluoride is in most toothpastes.** Commercial toothpastes contain many toxic additives. One of the worst is fluoride. If you look at the small print on the toothpaste, you will see the poison control warning, required by the F.D.A. Propylene glycol is another common toothpaste additive that has been associated with organ toxicity.[152] It poisons your sex organs and retards development in children. They even put plastics in toothpaste.[153] Plastics are endocrine disruptors.[154] This means that they interfere with your hormones. Knowing how toxic it is, there is no need to ever buy toothpaste again. It is much better to just make your own. You can just mix baking soda with Kosher salt (no additives). Put the mix in a little bowl next to your toothbrush and dip your brush in it.

## Consider the balance of good to bad "bugs."

**The gut and the mouth are intimately connected.** Many of us understand that health begins in the gut. What many of us do not know is that the cornerstone of health is in the mouth and that the balance of good to bad microorganisms that live in the mouth is just as important as it is in the gut.

**The bacteria that are found in your mouth and gut create the microbiome.** Microbes work as symbiotic organisms to support you. The microbes are an important part of your immune system. The mouth and gut are both parts of the Gastrointestinal (G.I.) system needing good bacteria to control the bad bacteria. The G.I. tract begins in the mouth. The mouth is the second largest reservoir of bacteria. Only the lower G.I. tract is home to more bacteria than the mouth. Researchers have identified over 700 bacterial species in the mouth.[155] Some of these bacteria are directly associated with the development of diseases, like various forms of arthritis. When bad bacteria overcome the good bacteria in the mouth or the gut, our health suffers. Just as we should establish good gut bacteria to improve the health of our immune system, it is just as important to maintain the right balance of good to bad bacteria in the mouth.

**Probiotics are the types of microbes that help you.** They produce Vitamin K and enzymes and crowd out bad bacteria that can cause tooth decay and periodontal disease. When we have an unhealthy diet, we attract the bad bacteria, which can overwhelm the good bacteria. Good probiotics can restore a healthy balance. The healthy microbiome has plenty of good bacteria that work in your behalf to help your health. The problems come in when you have an overgrowth of the bad bacteria like strep or E.coli.

**Taking antibiotics is a real insult to building a healthy microbiome.** Rampant antibiotic use is wrecking the microbiome. This is a major cause of tooth decay. Even toothpaste contains antibiotics that kill off the good bacteria and disturb the balance of the microbiome. GMO's, preservatives, food additives, vaccinations (flu shots), and nutrient-poor foods contribute to a body that is toxic and under-nourished. Then we become susceptible to all manner of disease from autism to Alzheimer's.[156] If you do all of the right things, you can improve your microbiome rapidly. If you are very diligent, really cleaning up your act, you could improve your microbiome in as little as a few months. Learn to make cultured vegetables, yogurt, kefir, and other cultured foods and eat them at every meal.

## Mouthwashes that kill.

New studies are now finding that mouthwash use is associated with increased risk of head and neck cancers.[157] [158] When deciding what to use to rinse out your mouth, follow this advice, "If you would not eat or drink it because it is a poison, it is not smart to rinse your mouth with it." Using any toxic chemicals in the mouth poisons your whole body. Everything that touches your mouth or other skin is absorbed into your body. Re-evaluate all of your personal care products with this in mind, especially skin products.

Better choices are natural substances, like essential oils, oil pulling,[159] or herbs that you wouldn't be afraid to swallow. In the 19th century, the mouthwash, Listerine®, was made from four essential oils. Later, the oils were replaced by alcohol and other chemicals that may burn your gums.[160] We may be served better to go back to the original idea and use essential oils as a mouthwash, rather than using products that contain alcohol and other harmful chemicals.

Many popular mouthwashes and dental treatments contain chlorhexidine, which kills the good bacteria in your microbiome, raising blood pressure.[161] The good bacteria play an important role in keeping your blood pressure at a healthy level.[162] Chlorhexidine has been proven to raise blood pressure, increasing your risk of heart attack and stroke.[163] [164] Patients suffering from gingivitis and dental plaque are usually treated with topical antimicrobials, such as Corsodyl or Peridex mouthwash, of which the active ingredient is chlorhexidine. Triclosan is another toxic agent in dental therapy used as an antimicrobial. It has also been widely used as a pesticide since the 60's. It has been shown to harm kidney function.[165]

## Detoxify.

**Prevention is just as important for your own health as it is for the health of your car.** Detoxification of your body is just as important for your own health as getting an oil change is for your car. Proper nutrition with plenty of fiber is important. Do everything you can to prevent the toxins from coming into your body. Get a HEPA air filter. Filter your drinking and bathing water. Avoid personal care products and cleaning products with toxic chemicals. Avoid toxic dental materials.

Clean your colon. A bowel movement every day is essential to detoxify. If you don't have frequent bowel movements, toxins are just sitting there, being absorbed back into the system. You end up with malabsorption and toxicity. Bentonite clay, 1/4 to 1/2 teaspoon a day, will bind the toxins until you evacuate. Mix it with food if you feel toxic. Master cleanses, Perfect 7, bentonite, magnesium flushes, saltwater flushes, coffee enemas, and the like will keep the colon clean. If you are losing weight or getting mercury fillings removed, it is especially important to cleanse the colon. Mercury can lodge in the nervous system during mercury detoxification if mercury levels get too high during detoxification. When you lose weight, toxins that were stored in the fat tissues come out into the bloodstream. Fasting or weight loss is necessary for health, but protect your kidneys. Also make sure the liver has all of the nutrients to process the toxins. Cleaning the liver on a regular basis gets the toxins out. The liver-gall bladder cleanse is the big gun.

Breathe clean air by walking in parks or woods. Use pranayama (yoga breathing) or other breathing exercise.

Get an inexpensive Far Infrared (FIR) sauna and use it every day. We have a small, collapsible FIR sauna, with FIR panels on the walls and a ceramic heater.

After getting the toxic metals removed from your mouth, you may decide to get tested for heavy metals to determine the degree of your toxic burden. Then you can see the extent of the problem. A holistic dentist or physician can order the tests for you. Our book, "Secrets to Lose Toxic Belly Fat,"[166] discusses testing and treatment plans in detail. Detoxification that is too aggressive may cause severe damage, especially to the kidneys. This is why it is important to work with a holistic physician or biological dentist who understands how to detox safely, at a manageable pace, improving liver and kidney function to open up the pathways of detoxification. It may take a year or more of detoxification to safely detox from toxic heavy metals like mercury.

# 7. GUM DISEASE.

**Half of us have gum disease!** Almost one in two Americans over the age of 30 has periodontal disease.[167] This is an embarrassing statistic because periodontal disease is a preventable disease. It is the most common disease of all. And 11% of all people worldwide have SEVERE gum disease.[168]

**Symptoms of gum disease:**
- Redness in the gums.
- Gums that feel or look inflamed.
- Gums that bleed when you brush or floss.
- Teeth are loose.
- Pockets in the gums indicating bone loss.
- Bad breath.
- Gum disease is often silent, like heart disease or diabetes in the initial stages. There may be no symptoms. No pain or bleeding.

**Smoking quadruples your chances of losing your teeth.** 90% of those with severe gum disease are smokers.[169]

**Gum disease is preventable.** Brushing properly, flossing, using an irrigation device, regular holistic dental cleaning and check-ups are the key habits that prevent periodontal disease. Proper nutrition is essential to healing gum disease. You need to get enough vitamins and minerals and protein. Deficiencies in the diet are reflected in gum health.

**Gum disease equals chronic disease and tooth loss.** If left untreated, this chronic inflammatory condition that affects the gums and bones supporting the teeth, can lead to tooth loss and many kinds of chronic diseases. The inflammation in the gums is reflected in tissues all over the body.[170] [171] [172] It works the other way around, too. Illness in other parts of the body affects the health of the gums.

**The bacteria that cause gum disease are found in the arteries of people with heart disease.**[173] [174] Gum disease significantly increases risk for stroke.[175] Gum disease also increases risk for diabetes (and vice-versa),[176] rheumatoid arthritis,[177] and oral cancer.[178] In pregnant women, it causes an increase in risk for pre-term birth.[179] Medical doctors are beginning to understand this relationship. If they see a high level of white blood cells in the patient's blood, they may suspect periodontal disease, and refer the patient to a dentist who can examine them.

**Gum disease (periodontal disease) now causes more teeth to be lost than tooth decay.** As the disease progresses, the gums recede, exposing the roots of the teeth. Pockets of infection under the gum line increase, which leads to bone loss. As bone loss progresses, the teeth are not supported properly, leading to loose teeth. This is a dangerous cycle that makes it harder to keep the teeth clean, leading to loss of those teeth.

**Many think that gum disease is genetic, because their parents had it.** This is not entirely true. Most people have it, so the chances are high that their parents had it, too. You may have a genetic weakness, but it is your environment and lifestyle that may cause the disease to express itself.

**The conventional approach is poisoning us.** The advice given to us by conventional dentists about healing periodontal disease does not work and is downright dangerous. Natural therapies, such as using essential oils, are not even considered by most dentists.

**Do not get your teeth cleaned until you are sure that you do not have a gum infection.** Just because your dentist has you rinse your mouth out with mouthwash before a cleaning doesn't mean that the cleaning will be safe. The mouthwash itself may be a toxic concoction. When you go to the dentist, insist on getting the check-up first, to determine that you do not have a gum infection, before getting your teeth cleaned. This is especially important if you have a heart valve murmur, a weak pancreas, or arthritis. When you have eradicated the infection and the microscopic slide shows that you are clear, then you can get your teeth cleaned. A disinfection and laser-type of cleaning is safer than ordinary teeth cleaning.

**Gum disease is caused by microorganisms in our mouths that can be seen under the microscope.**[180] The dentist scrapes a bit of plaque off of the tooth under the gum line, puts it on a slide under the phase contrast microscope and examines the bacteria found in the plaque to determine whether the problem is bacterial, fungal, or parasites. Viruses are not usually the cause. If the dentist sees huge swarms of bugs, looking like traffic jams on the freeway in L.A. at rush hour, you have a problem. If there are only a few bugs, looking like the number of cars on a lonely stretch of road at 3 am, then you do not have a problem. When the bad bugs that are causing the infection are eradicated, the gum disease can be halted.

**Once we have identified a harmful micro-organism, we then decide how to get rid of it.** If you can kill the infection without antibiotics, that is the best choice. Herbs may do the trick. But if the infection is severe, herbal protocols may be too slow, and you may have to resort to prescription drugs.

**Bacterial infections are the easiest to treat because they can be treated topically.** Harder to treat are the people who have lost a lot of bone, that really bleed, have terrible bad breath, and those who have parasites.

**Most dentists are not prepared to treat parasitic infections.** The amoeba is one parasite that many of us live with.[181] It destroys our gums. It feeds on the white blood cells and takes the hemoglobin out of our red blood cells. This is a challenge to our immune system and makes us feel tired. The most common parasite causing gum disease is the amoeba, Entamoeba gingivalis. It is not just found in the mouth, but throughout the entire body. You may need to see a physician who understands how to effectively diagnose and treat parasites. See our book, "Secrets to Lose Toxic Belly Fat" to learn more about diagnosing and treating parasites.[182]

**Methods of treating parasites:**
- Herbal parasite cleanses include a black walnut tincture and aloe vera, which are anti-bacterial, anti-fungal, and anti-parasitic.
- Ozone is a potent natural substance, but is difficult to use because it is toxic when you breathe it.
- MMS is a disinfectant that works.
- Diatomaceous earth.
- Essential oils.
- Bentonite clay.
- Hot salt water.
- Oil pulling.
- Chewing on cloves.
- Metronidazole is commonly used to kill parasites. The problem with strong drugs like this is that the liver must work very hard to get rid of them. Sometimes though, this may be the better choice. Speak with your doctor and get his or her advice.

The problem with many of these methods is that they won't kill the parasites all over the body. These methods may only work to kill parasites in the mouth. The parasites come back because they are still living in the colon. You may have to resort to powerful drugs to completely eliminate parasites.

**Gum disease may continue to spread among family members, until all family members have been treated.** Even pets can spread their gum disease to the members of their human family. So, if you want to stay free of gum infections, don't forget to treat your pets and all family members at the same time that you are being treated.

**Gum problems also have other causes.** Perhaps the microscopic evaluation does not reveal a lot of bacteria, but you are still having problems with your gums. Some medications may cause gum problems.[183] Swollen, puffy, fragile gums, and dry mouth are side effects of some medications. This may make it too painful or difficult to care for your gums properly. Consult with your doctor if you are experiencing gum problems that might be caused by medications. If your hormones are unbalanced or deficient, your gums will also tell the story.

## The alternative to gum surgery.

**One of the caveats of medicine is, "Do not cut into tissue that is infected."** For instance, doctors do not remove tonsils when they are actively infected. Yet this rule is often ignored in dentistry. Dentists may cut on gums that are bleeding or exuding pus. Unfortunately, in most general dental offices, this is the first thing that they do. If a dental cleaning is done before the first check-up, it could be spreading the disease straight into the bloodstream, and into the rest of the body. "Cut and sew" surgical procedures are often painful, require weeks of healing, and are usually ineffective at curing periodontal disease in the long term.

### To heal your gums without surgery:

(1) Remove pathogens. This will usually require 3-5 visits to the biological dentist to complete. The entire mouth is irrigated with an antimicrobial rinse that contains essential oils and herbs to reduce pathogens going into the blood stream before periodontal therapy begins. Then the periodontal pockets are treated. Natural antibiotics like garlic extract or oil of oregano are used to rinse the mouth to treat inflammation and infection.

(2) Balance your body chemistry. To make your body more alkaline, increase the amounts of fruits and vegetables consumed and cut out processed food and grains.

(3) Get regular hygiene check-ups, every 3 – 4 months at first, then increase to 6 months as appropriate for your individual situation.
- Continue to follow your strict program of brushing, flossing, and Water Pik usage.
- Eat a healthy diet.
- Take nutritional supplements.

### The trouble with pockets.

Bacteria that are allowed to remain in the mouth from lack of proper dental hygiene flourish in an acidic environment, causing inflammation of the gums and bone loss surrounding the teeth. These bacteria create periodontal pockets in the bone that are measured in millimeters by dental probing and are difficult to clean properly. The ideal measurement is between one and three millimeters. When you get above a three, you have lost some of the attachment and bone around the teeth. When you get up at seven and above, you really cannot effectively clean the pockets at home, even with a Water Pik.

If not corrected, more dangerous bacteria invade the periodontal pockets. Their by-products accelerate the bone loss and inflammation of the gums. This process can develop painlessly until the inflammation is trapped between the gum and the tooth causing an abscess or pocket of pus. The pus is made up of dead white blood cells the body has sent out to fight the infection. As the pus ball enlarges, the gum becomes tender. The infection can spread and seem like it is going into your ear or under your lower jaw and down into your neck. It may become hard to open your mouth because of swelling.

The usual dental method of relieving this "periodontal abscess" is to prescribe medications such as Amoxicillin or Erythromycin to control the infection and prevent seeding into the heart and blood vessels. The gum area of the periodontal pocket will be cleaned out of debris and the pus drained by the dentist. This will alleviate most of the immediate pain. However, the underlying problem still remains and without further treatment, it will happen again.

### Tough infections respond to this.

**Ozonated olive oil is a safe, effective alternative to conventional medications.** Studies show that it works even better than chlorhexidine and povidone-iodine at killing common gum infections.[184] The use of ozonated olive oil for gum pockets can be extremely helpful. Ozonated oil is inexpensive and will last indefinitely when refrigerated. The use of ozonated olive oil for periodontal abscess is just beginning to be discovered. Alternative dentists who were working with ozone for dentistry discovered the value of ozonated oil for periodontal pockets and abscesses five years ago.

Ozonated olive oil is extra virgin olive oil that has had strong medical grade ozone bubbled through it for at least a month. High quality ozonated-oil manufacturers ozonate the oil for at least three months. It has a very thick consistency when refrigerated.

**48    TOXIC TEETH**

Ozonated oil is saturated with "ozonides." Ozonides have active oxygen in the molecule. Ozonated olive oil slowly releases this active oxygen, which inactivates viruses, destroys anaerobic bacteria, and also kills protozoa, yeast, and a host of other harmful organisms.

Daily use will destroy sufficient numbers of the bacteria to prevent colonization of the bacteria, reducing bone loss and inflammation.[185] Because it takes 24 hours of incubation of bacteria in a periodontal pocket for the organism to colonize to the point of causing destruction of bone or gum inflammation, ozonated olive oil should be used daily after a thorough cleaning of the teeth, gums and perio pockets. You can put it on your gums right before you go to sleep at night for maximum absorption. The ozonated olive oil can be applied with a toothbrush or with the tip of a finger to the gums. The oil will penetrate below the gums into perio pockets as deep as 9 mm.

Ozonated oil is also helpful in healing surgical wounds of the gums.[186] When combined with a mineral wash containing calcium sodium phosphosilicate, ozonated oil also helps to reverse the sensitivity in the dentin of the tooth after surgery.[187]

## How to clean teeth and gums properly.

**Make sure to get your teeth cleaned at least every six months by a good dental hygienist.** Get your teeth cleaned after the dentist has evaluated your mouth. Your dental team can help you to catch gum disease early, before it causes problems. They can also do deeper cleanings than you can, getting below the gum line to places you cannot reach. Your team can also educate you in how to prevent the build-up of the high-risk bacteria that cause gum disease. A good dental team will help you to prevent the progression of gum disease, so that no more bone is lost.

**Our goal is to remove the bad bacteria and their hiding places.** If you let the plaque build up, it will turn into calculus. Then your hygienist will have to remove it.

### 1. Brush properly.

**Use a soft bristle brush.** Aim the brush at the gum line. Angle the brush up into the gums for upper teeth, down for lower teeth. Don't saw away with the brush. That can damage the gums. Use only gentle pressure, jiggling, and circular motion for a few seconds. An electric toothbrush can be very helpful, because the motor does the jiggling work for you. Work on one tooth at a time, pick up the brush and go to the next spot. Don't miss the back sides of the teeth. Every surface needs to be brushed. Spend a few seconds on the inside of each tooth of the lower jaw, then a few seconds on the inside of each tooth on the upper jaw. Then brush for a few seconds on each tooth on the outside of the lower jaw and then brush for a few seconds on the outside of each tooth of the upper jaw. You need to be very systematic. Count one one hundred, two one hundred, three one hundred on each tooth before moving on. Brushing your teeth this way should take you about three to five minutes.

If you have gum disease, you can help yourself by spending a lot of spare time working a dry brush into the gums. Dry brushing helps to break up the biofilm of germs (plaque), and to mix air into the gums. Most of the bad bacteria are anaerobic, and don't tolerate oxygen. The more air they are exposed to, the more you will kill. You may notice truck drivers or farmers at truck stops with toothpicks in their mouths. They are on to something. By absently working the toothpick into their gums as they drive, they are exposing the anaerobic bacteria in their gums to air and killing them off, preventing gum disease.

## 2. Floss.

You MUST floss and/or use interdental brushes! You have to clean the area between the teeth just as diligently as you do the rest of the gums and teeth.

## 3. Irrigate the pockets.

A brush and floss will only reach about a millimeter into the crevice. To get under the gums more thoroughly, use an irrigator, like a Water Pik, to flush under the gums with a disinfecting solution. Use the rubber-tip attachment made for pockets. It shoots a gentle stream of water under the gums to clean pockets really well. This is not painful or, if it is, that is where the pocket of infection is located.

### What to put into your Water Pik: Any of these will work.
- Salt water. Do not use sea salt. Dr. Hal Huggins recommended Morton's pickling and canning salt because it has no additives.
- Diluted hydrogen peroxide (half-half water) if there are no amalgams.
- Salt water with a few drops of iodine (Betadine).
- Water with ozone bubbled through it from an ozone generator. Ozone water is antibacterial, antiviral, and antifungal.
- Herbal formulas.
- Diluted apple cider vinegar.
- Baking soda diluted in water.
- Powdered Vitamin C (sodium ascorbate).

## 8. ROOT CANALS: SOURCES OF INFECTION.

**A root canal is a procedure that is done most often when an infection from a cavity has gotten so deep that it has invaded the pulp tissue (the inside center portion of the tooth).** This inside center portion of the tooth is the root canal space. It contains the blood vessels and nerves of the tooth.

**Once the inside part of the tooth becomes infected, the tooth is filled with pus, and this must be drained.** The infection is killing the tooth and must be treated.

**The tooth must either be extracted or have a root canal.** When the inside part of the tooth becomes infected, the patient will feel pain in the tooth (like sensitivity to hot or cold, and sensitivity to pressure). The pain is usually quite severe. The dentist can see changes on the X-ray. That means that the bone around the tooth has been resorbed by the infection. When the dentist sees the X-ray changes, it is a definitive signal that action must be taken. When that pulp has become infected and died, the dentist will usually perform a root canal.

To do a root canal, the dentist first removes all the decay that caused the infection. The dentist then inserts a long barbed drill into the root canal all the way from the top of the tooth down into the root in an attempt to remove the infected tissue and widen and shape the canal space. The dentist will use larger and larger files, scraping the walls of the root canal. To kill the bacteria that have infected the tooth, an anti-microbial agent is inserted into the root canal. After doing his or her best to widen, shape and sterilize the canal, the space is sealed. The dentist then fills the middle of the tooth with a rubber-like material.

**The rest of the tooth can then fill up with bacteria or mold, sort of like the junk that grows on the grout in your shower.** Black scuzzy bacteria or mold can grow around the tooth. The gum tissue around the infected tooth starts to turn purple as the body tries to wall off this infection. It isn't pink like the tissue around a healthy tooth. It turns darker and more purplish, as the swelling in the tissue inhibits the blood flow in the veins.

**When the root-canal tooth is pulled, it smells terrible.** The smell starts to die down after a while, but if the tooth is broken open, it will continue to smell really awful. These bugs smell very, very bad because they are anaerobic bacteria. They have been growing without oxygen. These bugs can go all over the body, into the heart, the skin, anywhere.

## A root canal cannot sterilize an infected tooth.

"Root canals are a zillion times worse than mercury fillings." (Dr. Hal Huggins)[188] A healthy tooth has a circulation system to keep a tooth healthy. The root structure has little tubules that push out fluid. The blood flow in a live tooth keeps bacteria out.

**We can't fight off infection in a root canal tooth, because there is no blood flow into the dead tooth.** Bacteria that are living in the gums around the tooth can easily go right inside the tooth. The tooth is infected immediately after the root canal procedure and becomes more and more infected as bacteria multiply with time. No matter how good the dentist may be, there will ALWAYS be some infection left in the tooth after the root canal procedure has been completed.

The canal that runs through the center of the tooth has many small tubules that come off the side. Those lateral branches can never be free of infection. There are so many tubules that, if the tubules of the tooth were laid out end to end, they would reach three miles in length. They are wide enough to harbor bacteria.

When the tooth becomes infected, the bacteria take up residence in these tubules, just like a sponge soaking up water. No instrument, no antimicrobial irrigation, no lasers, nothing can touch the bacteria living there in those tubules.

**Biological dentists insist that all root canal teeth are infected.** The rest of the dentists believe that infection is present in only a certain percentage of root canal teeth. In dental school, students are taught to keep irrigating and instrumenting the root canal until cultures done in the lab show no bacteria living in the canal space. Their belief is that when the culture comes back negative, the tooth can be safely sealed and the procedure completed. They believe that once the sealer is put into the root canal, any bacteria that are still there will become entombed and will not cause any further health problems. Both of these concepts are not based in fact.

**A dead tooth provides an immune system challenge.** A root canal is done to save a dead tooth. The body knows that the tooth is dead. The body tries to get rid of the dead tooth because it doesn't want it in your mouth. The immune system goes on overdrive to get rid of that dead tooth. If you have mercury fillings as well, the immune system is also under pressure from the mercury toxicity.

**The onset of a problem caused by a root-canal treated tooth happens when your immune system becomes compromised enough to allow disease to get started.**[189]

Many people have symptoms of disease that are related to the toxicity caused by root canals. Their bodies are incapable of detoxifying the poisons being produced by the root canal teeth. These people won't get better until the root canal teeth are properly removed.

Sure, maybe you can get away with no ill effects from one or two or maybe even three root-canal treated teeth when you are healthy at 20 or 30 years old. But as time goes on, these teeth become more infected, and the body experiences more health insults in the form of stress, accidents, toxicity from the environment, poor eating and sleeping habits, or whatever.

**Eventually a breaking point is reached and ill health results.** Some people can have a root canal for decades with no symptoms, because their bodies are very capable of handling toxicity. It's just like some people can smoke and drink and live to 100. But I wouldn't bet that I am one of those people.

**It is the combined assault that takes us down eventually.** The bacteria can travel to any organ in the body. We come down with sinus infections, emotional problems, asthma, or any one of a host of diseases. Root canal teeth may be the sources of infection that cause chronic inflammation all throughout the body, including the heart.[190][191] It is inflammation that causes a heart attack.

If this situation goes on long enough, your immune system becomes weakened and dysregulated and may not be able to protect you from diseases like cancer. Or it may become hyperactive. Then you get autoimmune diseases like allergies, asthma, Crohn's, ulcerative colitis, Hashimoto's Thyroiditis, rheumatoid arthritis,[192] etc.

Some root canals don't show any pathology on an ordinary dental X-ray. But this does not mean that they are not causing problems. In 1923, Dr. Weston Price,[193] a Cleveland dentist, informed us that the root canals that are causing the worst problems are often those that don't show any pathology on an X-ray.[194]

He surmised that the patient's immune system had not responded to the infection as it should, by forming an abscess around the tooth. This happens if a patient has a weakened immune system, especially if they are using a medication such as prednisone or methotrexate to treat auto-immunity. In these cases, the body will not form an abscess around the root-canaled tooth. The bacteria are free to flourish without being walled off by the immune system.

### *Should you get all root canals removed?*

**Realize that all root canal teeth will stay infected and get worse with time, negatively impacting your health.** If you value your health, don't get a root canal. If you have a root canal, it is important to deal with it by getting the correct procedure to have it removed.

**Don't ignore the immune system stress that is being caused by having a dead tooth in your mouth.** Sure, you may be able to handle the immune system stress for a while, or maybe you won't. But as you age and add other bodily insults, the immune system may eventually break down, and you may develop a disease as a result.

Regardless of whether you get a terrible disease or not, root canals and mercury fillings are harming your health. Your body can only suffer so many insults before it breaks down. Your mouth may be the site of the largest health insults of all.

## How root canals may affect your sinuses.

**When root canal treatment is performed on teeth with roots that are close to the maxillary sinus, it may cause big trouble.** Instruments and materials are frequently introduced beyond the end of the tooth (apical foramen) and into the maxillary sinus[195][196][197][198] harming the maxillary sinus.[199][200][201] After these accidents, patients report severe pain, edema, profuse bleeding, and sometimes secondary infection. The majority of cases showed complete resolution of symptoms within a couple of weeks. But a few had long-term abnormal sensation, such as burning, prickling, and a few had scarring.[202][203]

Even if all instrumentation is kept within the canal and there is no perforation into the sinus, some degree of inflammatory response normally occurs after root canal procedures.[204] Debris may migrate into the sinuses, causing inflammation, pain after the procedure, and delayed healing.[205][206] The sinus irritation may be so chronic and severe that a granuloma may form. If this gets worse, a cyst may form,[207] and this may progress to sinus bacterial infection.

In my 3D X-ray, a bubble above the root canal could be seen inside the sinus above it. It looked like the tooth was blowing a large bubble into the sinus. I sought out the most knowledgeable expert in cysts and periapical infections in my area. The oral surgeon told me that he sees these bubbles all the time and that they are harmless. The name he gave it was a "mucocele," the result of chronic inflammation at the apex of the maxillary root canal tooth.

## 9. JAWBONE CAVITATIONS.

**The jawbones (the maxilla above and mandible below) are more subject to infection and injury than any other bone.** When there is an injury, such as a root canal, an improperly-performed tooth extraction, infection after an extraction, or a blow to the jaw, the bone tissue in the jaw tends to have trouble healing. Even though the overlying gum tissue may look OK, a dead spot, or a hole may form in the jawbone. This is called jawbone osteonecrosis.[208]

**These dead spots or holes in the jawbones are known as cavitations.** Cavitations are areas of dead bone, filled with bacteria, and are highly toxic.

**Many people have undiagnosed cavitations, because they have jawbone infections but are not aware of them.** These infections are often silent and therefore difficult to find.

### Jawbone osteonecrosis is a silent disease caused by:
- Periodontal disease. As the disease progresses, the gums recede, exposing the roots of the teeth. Pockets of infection under the gum line increase, which leads to bone loss.
- Root canals.
- The use of epinephrine-containing local anesthetics used to stop bleeding during tooth extraction. This may result in dry socket.
- Trauma and infection.
- Bisphosphonates (like Fosamax, Boniva).[209][210][211][212] Researchers are studying treatment regimens, especially ozone,[213][214] for these patients.[215][216][217]
- Effects of certain medications[218] and recreational drugs.[219]
- Poor blood flow to the jaw (TMJ, diabetes, advancing age).
- Smoking (especially in the healing phase of tooth extraction).
- Alcoholism.
- Estrogen therapy or pregnancy.
- Corticosteroid therapy.
- Autoimmune diseases.
- Malnutrition (starvation, anorexia).
- Anemia.
- Radiation and chemotherapy.
- Metastatic cancer.
- Hypothyroidism.
- Genetic predisposition.[220]
- Reduced immune function.[221]

**Cavitations form most often where wisdom teeth have been removed, but are also found where any other teeth have been extracted.**[222] These areas of decayed, infected, abscessed bone tissue also often appear around a root-canaled tooth.

Root canals are always infected, and it is best to have them removed. When a tooth is infected, the bone around it is also infected. When that tooth is removed, it is important to address the issue of the infection in the jawbone, so that a smoldering infection is not left there. If any infection is left in the jawbone, that infection may cause disease in the body far from the mouth.[223]

In a cavitation, bone tissue has died and decayed, because blood and lymphatic circulation has been cut off. If all of the infection in the tooth socket is not removed, the site may become a breeding ground for bacteria that can invade the surrounding bone as well as the rest of the body, leading to serious health problems. The patient may end up with a festering bone that never gets well and may produce chronic, disabling pain in the jaw. If a nerve becomes impacted by a cavitation, it may cause jaw pain, facial pain, and the very painful facial pain of trigeminal neuralgia,[224] also known as tic douloureux.

**Many kinds of anaerobic bacteria live in these jawbone cavitations.** The toxins produced by these anaerobic bacteria in cavitations are among the most potent toxins known to mankind. These anaerobic bacteria and their toxins are risk factors for disease all over the body.[225][226][227] Cavitations can lead to cancer,[228][229] and other serious health issues.[230]

**Rectifying cavitations can dramatically improve your health.** Dramatic health improvements are not uncommon after a cavitation has been properly cleaned out, so that the source of disease is removed.[231] To have the cavitation surgery performed properly, find a biological dentist who has completed specific courses in order to learn how to properly extract teeth and how to clean out the sites of incorrectly extracted teeth.

### Symptoms that disappear after cavitation surgery:
- Chronic fatigue.
- Brain fog.
- Autoimmune symptoms.
- Trigeminal neuralgias.[232]
- Unexplained rashes and unexplained inflammatory issues.

**Cavitations have been acknowledged for centuries.** Also known as Cavitational Osteonecrosis, Ischemic Osteonecrosis,

NICO's,[233] [234] and various other labels, the presence of "necrotic," or dying bone in the jawbones has been discussed since the 1860's.[235] [236] G.V. Black's 1915 textbook devoted an entire section to the appearance and treatment of jawbone osteonecrosis.[237] More modern dental textbooks also discuss the issue.[238]

Research strongly supports the existence of jawbone cavitations. In a study of over 500 cavitations, it was found that over 75% are completely hollow or filled with soft, grayish-brown and mushy tissue, often with yellowish oily material.[239] [240] Others report cavitations lined with fibrous black, brown or grey filamentous materials,[241] with a texture that is "gritty", "like sawdust," and "dry," similar to the necrosis in other bones of the body.[242]

## Cavitations that cause facial pain.

**Cavitations that cause facial pain are called NICO.**[243] NICO stands for Neuralgia-Inducing Cavitational Osteonecrosis. Infections in the jawbone may cause demyelination of the nerve fibers. This means that the nerve fibers lose their protective coating. When this happens, it causes trigeminal neuralgia, a terrible facial pain that feels like an intermittent stabbing for five or so minutes.[244] Others with NICO don't have facial pain, but do have pain somewhere else, ankles, knees, low back, etc. This is called silent NICO.

Many people with trigeminal neuralgia have had success with healing their condition when they have had their jawbone cavitations cleaned out.[245] [246] Dentist, John Ahearne, reported that 450 patients suffering from Trigeminal Neuralgia received cavitation clean-out. After the treatment almost 94% of his patients experienced significant improvement, if not total abatement of their pain.[247] In another study of 190 patients who had cavitation surgery to resolve the pain of NICO, more than two thirds experienced complete or almost complete disappearance of neuralgic pain immediately or shortly after cleaning out their jawbone cavitations. The long-term abatement of neuralgic pain was total or almost total in 74% of treated patients.[248]

## Extraction techniques may cause cavitations.

Cavitations can develop where any tooth has been removed. Cavitations can be prevented if the dentist follows a strict protocol.

**This protocol includes removal of the periodontal ligament.** When the periodontal ligament (ligament connecting tooth to bone) is removed along with the tooth, bone cells from each side of the bone in the socket will grow to meet each other to complete healing.

## TOXIC TEETH

**After extracting a tooth, many dentists neglect to remove the periodontal ligament that holds the tooth in place.** When the periodontal ligament is left intact after an extraction, it will die, leaving dead tissue at the base of the tooth. This turns into a big party for the bugs. If you have been on antibiotics for the infected tooth, only the bad boys will be left. This may prevent bone healing in the socket where the tooth was removed.[249] If the periodontal ligament is not removed, a cap of bone only one to three millimeters thick will form over the top of the socket. This leaves a hole about the size of the root underneath this thin cap. It may fill with a gooey substance. The lining of the space becomes filled with inflammatory cells that contribute to autoimmune disease.

**A cavitation may also result when a dentist uses a local anesthetic with epinephrine.** The best option is to skip the epinephrine when you get a tooth extracted. You want to get a good blood flow and a good clot to form in the extraction site. The epinephrine causes constriction of the blood vessels. Your heart beats faster. You don't get much bleeding. This is good for the dentist because the patient stays numb for one or two hours and bleeding is slowed. But you don't get a good clot to form. As the small capillaries close, red blood cells cannot be delivered to the area. The bone cells are deprived of oxygen. When bone cells are deprived of oxygen for as little as 34 seconds, they will die. The bone cannot heal because it is dead. If you had four wisdom teeth taken out with epinephrine, it is a given that you now have four cavitations in the bone where the wisdom teeth roots used to be.

### A dry socket leads to cavitations.

**A dry socket occurs when you have a tooth extracted, the blood clot is lost, and the socket becomes inflamed.** Dry socket is the most common complication of tooth extraction. Dry socket can be generally avoided by going in after the tooth is extracted and scraping away any soft and mushy diseased tissue and putting multiple anti-microbials into the hole in the bone. A dry socket is a major cause for cavitations, or bone infections. Be careful not to disturb the clot. Do not smoke within 24 hours at least after the surgery. Smoking can cause a dry socket. Also do not drink through a straw or poke around the blood clot with your tongue.

### Root canals cause cavitations.

A root canal kills the tooth by removing the nerve/pulp from the root chamber and filling it with a latex and/or heavy metal-laden material. As the blood and lymph circulation ceases, the bone tissue becomes starved for oxygen, then dies, and eventually forms a cavitation. The dead bone tissue prevents the re-growth of healthy bone tissue, because the circulation can't get to it. The cavitation may then become infected or abscessed. Many times there is no pain, due to the absence of the tooth nerve and the tooth being dead, until infection builds up and the tooth becomes sensitive.

## General guidelines for extraction:

- Anesthetics that contain epinephrine should only be used when restriction of the blood flow is required. We want to keep the blood flowing freely to prevent bone cell damage, and prevent the formation of a dry socket.
- The tooth should be removed with as little trauma as possible.
- Biopsies should be taken from the base of the tooth socket to find out what bacteria are there and examined under a microscope.
- Infected bone from between teeth and the entire perimeter of the sockets should be removed. The ligament that held the tooth into the socket must be removed. This removes infected bone and allows proper healing, so the body can form new bone immediately.
- Proper antibiotics must be administered to kill the bacteria found in the biopsies.
- Use probiotics following the antibiotics.

## Health problems healed with cavitation treatment.

**Many health problems may respond to treatment of cavitations in the jaw.** Here are some anecdotal reports:[250]

- A man reports that he had limped and experienced debilitating chronic pain in his left hip for four years. After cavitation surgery, he is nearly pain free and the limp is intermittent.
- One lady reported that she had experienced chest pains and pain in her left arm for over two and a half years. Following cavitation surgery on three wisdom tooth sites, she was pain free.
- Another lady reported dramatic health improvement and welcome weight gain after the removal of a piece of root, a piece of amalgam, and the surrounding diseased jawbone at an extraction site of 20 years ago.
- Another patient reported that, after cavitation surgery on one site, tonsil and kidney pain ceased.

- A man was losing his eyesight and suffering from unbearable pain in the left eye. Three days after cavitation surgery on six sites, his eyesight cleared and the pain stopped.
- Suzie had been sick on and off for several years with fatigue, low immune system function, and other aches, pains, headaches, and general unwellness. Three months after cavitation surgery, her health had improved dramatically. She feels that the cavitation surgery was the turning point for her.[251]
- Before cavitation surgery, Patty had a suppressed immune system and Lyme's disease. She couldn't seem to recover from illness. The benefits to Patty are that she has not had any of the brain fog or dizziness that she used to get and does not have to rely on coffee to get going. She says that now she can walk to the park a few blocks from her home. She had not been able to walk there in over 2 years.[252]
- Ericka says that after her cavitation surgery the ringing in her ears that had been present for six years subsided. She also said that she could hear better out of her left ear.[253]

## Should you be concerned about cavitations?

**Cavitations don't always cause problems that bother people.** Many people with cavitations go through their whole lives with no problems. Their bodies are able to handle the challenges caused by the dead bone in their jaws with no symptoms whatsoever. Others cannot handle the challenge of the toxicity being produced by the pathogens in the dead bone in their jaws.

It is just like any other health challenge. Some people can smoke two packs of cigarettes a day for decades, no problem. For others, just the smell of cigarette smoke precipitates an asthma attack. We are all different in our responses to health challenges.

And someone who is healthy at one point in time may be pushed over the edge into illness at another point in the future. At this point, the challenge of cavitations, root canals, and toxic fillings, combined with all of the other health challenges of life, may become too much for the body to handle. Then each dental issue becomes a serious contributor to illnesses.

If you are not experiencing any health problems, diagnosing and treating cavitations may be very low on your personal to-do list. But if you do have illness with no obvious cause, it may be wise to get a 3D jaw X-ray and send it to a biological dentist for evaluation.

**Cavitations in your mouth may be part of the cause or even the primary driver behind your diseases.** The immune system can only put up with so much toxicity. Then illness results. Many people experience health improvement when they get their cavitations cleaned out by a competent biological dentist.

**On the other hand, you may be barking up the wrong tree.** Cavitations may only play a minor or no role at all in your illness. If that is the case, you could be wasting a lot of money treating cavitations, not to mention the pain involved in healing from them. It may take up to six months to fully recover from jawbone surgery to clean out cavitations.

**It may be dangerous to assume that you do not have jawbone disease.** Most jawbone lesions are difficult to diagnose with routine radiographs and most are not painful.[254] This does not mean that jawbone disease does not exist. Many diseases are difficult to diagnose and many are not painful. This includes early stages of gum disease, diabetes, and most cancers.

**If you have jawbone infections, you need to find a skilled dentist to clean out the infected areas.** The problem is that there are very few dentists who are aware of this common condition. Treating silent bone infections is not taught in dental school and has been labeled as a controversial procedure by the dental profession. That is why you will need to visit a biological dentist.

The most difficult question to answer is, "Are the cavitations silent but significant or silent and insignificant?" This is why it is advisable to get a 3D X-ray and send it off to some biological dentists to get their expert opinions.

### Cavitation surgery may have to be repeated.

**Sometimes patients may have to return for another treatment on a cavitation that was already treated.** Bill talks about his own experience with facial pain and cavitations in an internet blog.[255] After routine dental treatment in his lower jaw, irritation developed in that area. Treatments from a dentist, an endodontist, and an oral surgeon exacerbated the pain. Bill was referred to a neurologist who diagnosed atypical trigeminal neuralgia. Over the next year, he suffered from serious pain.

Cavitation surgery was long, but tolerable. Recovery took place over a few months with gradual steady improvement. He became pain-free without medication. Three years later neuralgia-like pain returned to the lower jaw. The cavitation surgery was repeated. The procedure again resulted in remission of pain. For the next several years, he was free of jaw pain without medication. But then, after dental crown treatment, the pain returned to the lower jaw.

## Treatment modalities that reduce cavitation recurrence.

**The cavitation recurrence rate drops in direct proportion to the skill of the dentist and the treatment modalities used.** Do your homework before choosing a dentist to clean out your cavitations. Choosing a dentist who is recommended by Huggins Applied Healing will reduce your chances of needing to get the cavitation surgery repeated. Call 1-866-948-4638 for a current list of Huggins-trained dentists. These dentists have been thoroughly trained to do the procedure with a high level of expertise.

**They also use the latest treatment modalities to ensure success of the treatment.** Using platelet-rich plasma and platelet-rich fibrin reduces the need for repeat surgeries.[256] Using conscious sedation is probably worth the extra expense, because you won't have to experience the trauma of holding your mouth open for a long period of time. The reduced trauma may allow quicker healing time. Many patients' stories about cavitation surgery involve the trauma of shots and pain from holding their mouths open when not under sedation.

I had my cavitation surgery six months ago. I have had complete remission of the eye pain I was experiencing. It is my opinion that the skill of the dentist, ozone, PRF, intravenous Vitamin C, and conscious sedation are of major importance in reducing the necessity of repeated treatments.

## Identifying cavitations.

**Dental history will tell you a lot about whether or not you have cavitations.** Did you ever have a dry socket following an extraction? This is a dry bony wall without a blood clot in it. This is usually very painful. This almost always results in a cavitation.

The philosophy at Huggins Applied Healing is that any tooth that was removed with the periodontal ligament left in the mouth will be a candidate for a cavitation. Since most dentists do not remove the periodontal ligament when they extract a tooth, any extraction site would thus be a likely prospect for developing a cavitation. I had cavitations in my jawbones around every tooth I had ever had extracted.

**Dental cavitations cannot usually be detected by visual inspection.** Cavitations are difficult to diagnose, because they don't usually show on regular X-rays. It is difficult to see the wisdom teeth areas, where most of the pathologies exist. If you get pan-oral X-rays, where the X-ray machine rotates around the head, you may see changes in the bone where the wisdom teeth were removed. Because

**62   TOXIC TEETH**

40% or more of the bone needs to be altered to show changes on standard dental radiographs, the disease state is sometimes referred to as "undetectable" on ordinary dental films.[257] The first thing you do see is demineralization. This appears as a dark area.

### 3D X-rays more reliably detect cavitations.

**Because regular panoramic X-rays are not as reliable, newer scanners now can be utilized to find cavitations.** These include Tech 99 scans, MRI with filters, CAT scans, digital radiography, and "thru transmission ultrasonography" (Cavitat™).[258] The Cavitat™ ultrasound has been used for many years, but is no longer manufactured.

**3D X-rays more reliably reveal jawbone infections and bone loss.**[259] Cone-Beam Computed Tomography (CBCT) has proven to be a reliable method of identifying and estimating the size and extent of cavitations in the jaws.[260] You can view a place of interest in three dimensions using highly accurate measurement tools with advanced software.[261] [262] But, because most dentists and oral surgeons do not believe that jawbone infections exist, most are not interested in getting these expensive machines to detect them.

3D X-rays also may find malignant areas in wisdom-teeth infected areas.[263] [264] These 3D machines put out about twice the radiation of the traditional panoramic X-ray, so that is a concern. If the cavitations can be seen on the panoramic X-ray, you may not wish to expose yourself to more radiation by getting a 3D X-ray. Traditional panoramic X-rays along with a patient's history can be used to make a determination about whether or not surgery is advisable. Most dentists do not use this newer 3D technology yet. But if you choose to only get a 2D X-ray, you may be missing cavitations that could be found with a 3D X-ray.

**The interpretation of dental films is subjective.** Trained dentists may have different interpretations.[265] I sent my own 3D X-rays to four different biological dentists who specialize in cleaning out cavitations. Two agreed that I had nine cavitations. One said I had eight. And one said I had five. After further review, he revised that to eight. Two conventional dentists agreed that I had no cavitations.

### Diagnosing cavitations from symptoms.

**When infections in the jawbones are directly related to a symptom somewhere else in the body, the connection can be verified using a simple technique.** Using the dental meridian chart, a biological dentist can see if he can make the symptoms go away by injecting an anesthetic, like Novocain, into the cavitation site corresponding to the organ where the symptom is manifesting and see if the symptom goes away. [266]

Sam suffered from vertigo when reading. So the dentist had Sam read until he got vertigo and then injected some Novocain into the wisdom teeth area to see if his symptoms changed at all. The vertigo stopped immediately. Now that the source of the problem had been identified, the problem could be solved. Cleaning out the wisdom teeth cavitation sites cured Sam's vertigo completely.

If injecting a local anesthetic into the wisdom teeth areas gets rid of low back pain, cleaning out the jawbone infection may cure chronic low back pain. Heart problems may also be stemming from jawbone infection. Patients who are having a heart attack frequently report the pain radiating down the arm from the jaw. This may not be just a referred nerve pain. The patient may very likely have chronic infections in the wisdom teeth bone areas. An E.R. doctor might be able to avert a heart attack by injecting the wisdom teeth cavitation areas with Novocain.

## How to treat cavitations.

**There aren't many dentists who are prepared to treat cavitations, even if they knew how to diagnose them.** A dentist needs special training to learn how to do cavitation surgery properly. Biopsy to confirm the diagnosis of jawbone disease and rule out other disease states including cancer is important. Then, treatment to remove or eliminate the involved pathology and stimulate the regrowth of normal, vital bone is necessary.

Treatment requires removing dead bone and associated infection, using ozone and platelet-rich plasma (PRP) or platelet-rich fibrin (PRF), in order to restore good blood circulation and healthy bone in the area. PRP and PRF are made by centrifuging the patient's blood and drawing off the top layer. The use of PRF and PRP aid clotting and the release of growth factors over a period of up to fourteen days following surgery.[267] [268] [269] [270] [271]

Cavitation surgery is not considered to be a major surgery. After numbing the patient, the biological dentist makes an incision in the gums and pulls back a flap to expose the bone. He cracks out little windows in the bone to give him access to the soft inner bone. Then the dentist drills down to see if an oil-like substance oozes out. This is bone that has degenerated into fat. This is called saponification. The dead bone has literally degenerated into soap. He uses instruments to scrape out as much of the mushy dead bone as he can.

**The most important thing is to get all the dead bone out.** If the dentist doesn't get all the dead bone out, the surgery will fail. He puts the dead bone in a biopsy container to be analyzed. Then the dentist cleans down to the hard, bleeding bone and lets the void fill with blood. The dentist sterilizes the socket with as many as ten antimicrobials and ozone to kill the viruses and packs it with resorbable collagen material that has anti-microbials on it.

Healing is enhanced by inserting PRF or PRP grafts into the void. Other healing aids being used during and after cavitation surgery include intravenous high-dose Vitamin C, acupressure, homeopathy, electrical stimulation, radiation such as laser and infrared, medical grade oxygen/ozone, hyperbaric oxygen, anticoagulation modalities, nutrition and nutraceuticals, energy treatments, and others.

Finally, the dentist sews up the incision, and the wound is completely closed. The clot becomes fibrous and bony. Six months later it calcifies into normal alveolar bone. The patient will be sore for a week. Most patients require little or no pain medication.

**People usually report more energy, feeling better, with better overall health.** The symptoms caused by the cavitation usually go away and stay away for the rest of the patient's life. Facial neuralgias often clear up.[272] People's health usually improves when an infection anywhere in the body is cleaned up. Cleaning up the infections in cavitations is no different.

**Many of those afflicted with cavitations also have yeast infections,** both localized in the cavitations and systemically. The yeast infections are greatly increased when an antibiotic has been required to manage the tooth infection. One course of antibiotics, and your microbiome is forever changed. Following an anti-yeast diet is advisable.[273]

### Follow-up care.

Follow-up care may include remedies that encourage a good supply of blood, nutrients, and oxygen to re-grow the bone and good lymphatic drainage to remove toxins:
- Acupressure.
- Magnets.
- Ozonated olive oil.
- Ionized oxygen.
- Low-level healing laser therapy.
- Enzyme therapy.
- Homeopathic remedies.

## How conventional dentists treat cavitations.

**Most conventional dentists are resistant and sometimes even defensive about treating cavitations.** Even though cavitations are discussed in dental textbooks, and have been for many years, and are well-documented in all of the literature, dentists were not trained in dental school to identify and treat these lesions. The medical profession has been trained to identify and remove dead tissue anywhere in the body. But the dental profession has often ignored dead tissue when it is in the mouth.

When I questioned a prominent oral surgeon with 40 years of experience about his stance on cavitations, he replied that cavitations are best left undisturbed. In his opinion, cavitation surgery is opening a can of worms that may cause more problems down the line. I can understand why he said this. I certainly would not want an untrained dentist to perform cavitation surgery in my mouth. Only a very few dentists (biological) feel that cavitation surgery is warranted and have been trained to properly perform cavitation surgery.

If you have any of the risk factors for cavitations that we discussed earlier, get 3D X-rays and send them off for evaluation to some good biological dentists[274][275] who use intravenous Vitamin C, conscious sedation, and PRF or PRP. It is best not to allow any other dentists to perform cavitation surgery in your mouth.

## Replacing a lost tooth.

**To replace the lost tooth, the least invasive method is a removable appliance that you take in and out at will.** The artificial tooth is on a metal or plastic base. This is a partial denture, also called a removable bridge.

**The next option is a bridge.** You cap the tooth on either side of the missing tooth and cement an artificial tooth in between. This doesn't come out. The teeth on either side of the missing tooth must be ground away a bit in order to prepare the surface for the bridge supports. This does weaken these teeth somewhat.

Be careful not to use two different types of metals in the bridge. It may cause an unpleasant galvanic response.

**The most invasive option is a dental implant.** It is placed into the bone, simulating a tooth root. A hole is drilled into the jawbone. The implant is inserted into the bone. If you do decide to get an implant, be aware that ozonated oil may improve the quality of integration into the bone and may influence bone density[276] and decreased infection. You then usually wait for three to six months to get the implant to lock into the bone. You can get a crown made of zirconium or porcelain or another material of your choice. Zirconium is the most bio-inert material. A bio-compatibility test will determine which materials will work best for you.

**Are implants a safe replacement for teeth?** Although implants may enhance your appearance, you need to be aware that the use of any kind of implant may create other health challenges. For people who already have health challenges, it may be better to refuse to get implants of any kind.[277] At Huggins Applied Healing in Colorado Springs, they say that, "We have seen numerous diseases with an unknown origin that may have been created by implants."[278] More than a dozen different anaerobic bacteria have been found around implants that are supposedly healthy.[279]

I personally had a front upper tooth extracted and opted for a partial. I don't like the partial, because I find it to be uncomfortable. It does bind up my maxilla, which restricts the Cranialsacral rhythm. I only wear it on special occasions, as it is a front tooth. But I am glad that I did not opt for an implant. Dentists and hygienists continually urge me to get an implant. An implant might cause symptoms or not, but it is a foreign body and our bodies don't like foreign bodies. I just tell people that I have returned to the innocence of my 7-year old self with the missing front tooth.

In the U.S., about 99% of the dental implants placed are made of metal. Titanium alloys are titanium mixed with a number of other metals for strength. One of the metals alloyed with titanium is aluminum. The metal ions may travel throughout the body, increasing allergies. If you have a known metal allergy, you definitely would like to avoid metal implants. If you are considering a metal implant, it would be wise to get an allergy test for metals.[280] Years after getting a titanium implant in the mouth or the hip or someplace else, health may deteriorate. But rarely does anyone consider that the cause may be a reaction to the titanium implant. We just don't know what the long-term consequences are of getting a titanium implant. We know more about the short-term consequences (infection), because the implant is a foreign body. Why use metal implants when non-metal alternatives exist? Zirconium alloys are more bio-compatible than titanium alloys.

**If you wait long enough, there may be a protocol to grow back your own lost teeth using stem cells.**[281] It may happen within five or ten years or so. The technique will be to put collagen into the socket that will attract the stem cells to direct the growth of a brand new tooth![282] [283] I am not going to hold my breath waiting for this to happen, but when it does, I may consider it.

## 10. PROBLEMS WITH WISDOM TEETH.

**If your wisdom teeth erupt properly at the right time, you've got it made.** Leave them alone.[284] Getting these third molars removed may not seem like a big deal, but it is still an invasive technique. Every treatment has its risks. Infections, complications with anesthesia, or surgical complications are all possible. If the socket is not thoroughly disinfected, the development of cavitations is likely.

## Impacted wisdom teeth need to be extracted.

**If a wisdom tooth is impacted, it means that it is either not out fully or isn't in the position it should be.** If you have no more room in your mouth for the wisdom tooth, it will go sideways trying to find a way out and just end up impacted. Then you have to get it cut out rather than pulled.

**Some impacted teeth are laterally impacted.** They are lying on their side. Other impacted teeth are in the right position, with the crown up and the roots down, but something is preventing them from coming out.

When wisdom teeth are impacted, you have tissue that belongs on the outside of the body (the crown) inside the body. The body will not tolerate this. It hurts.

The first thing the body does is to send white blood cells in to dissolve the offending tissue (the crown of the tooth). If it can't dissolve it, it will put fluid around it, and you develop a cyst in the jawbone. This doesn't always happen. If the immune system doesn't work very well, the impacted tooth may just sit in the jawbone for years (as many as 30 years or so) before turning into a cyst. Dentists are trained to remove impacted teeth when they become cystic. But, if you wait for the impacted tooth to finally become cystic, you have to take it out right away, or you will have more problems.

**It is best to take the impacted tooth out immediately, before it becomes cystic.** You don't want to leave tissue that belongs on the outside of the body on the inside for any length of time. The body will use a lot of white blood cells trying to fight the problem.

An impacted wisdom tooth might not be painful right now, but later on it may cause problems. If the tooth is impacted, you have added stress to your immune system. The last thing you want is to add more stress to your immune system. Your immune system needs to deal with the other burdens in our toxic world. So, get any impacted wisdom teeth extracted.

## Improper extraction leads to bone loss.

**Bone loss usually begins in the wisdom area and then moves forward in the mouth, tooth by tooth, encompassing the molars and bicuspids.** This scenario might be prevented if the wisdom teeth were properly removed in the first place.

**The problem with wisdom teeth extraction is finding a good dentist who will do the job properly, so that bacteria don't cause a smoldering infection that persists decades later.** That smoldering infection causes diseases distant in the body from the mouth. A dentist is not usually consulted, because the connection between jawbone disease and other disease is not made. People end up seeing a specialist who knows nothing about the mouth.

**The wisdom teeth are connected to the heart by acupuncture meridians.** If your wisdom teeth were removed when you were 20, by the time you are 50, the toxins seeping out of the cavitations may cause heart problems. So it is best to have a biological dentist look at 3D X-rays of your mouth to see if you have cavitations around the sites of the wisdom teeth extractions. If you do have cavitations, getting them cleaned out may save you from heart disease and other health problems.

**When the wisdom tooth (or any other tooth) is taken out, it is important to completely remove the sack around the tooth (ligament that attached the tooth to the bone).** Hal Huggins comments on the importance of removing the periodontal ligament after extraction. "It takes only 3 or 4 minutes to remove the ligament after the surgery is completed, and could alleviate much pain and true agony of slow death from autoimmune diseases."[285]

## What happens in old extraction sites?

**What are the concerns around old extraction sites?** If the bone marrow never healed properly, you have infection and a site where toxins are being produced by pathogens.

Over fifty different anaerobic toxin-producing bacteria have been identified in cavitations.[286] When these toxins begin to seep out of cavitations, you have problems, because there is no circulation inside the cavitation. There may be pus or black junk in there. This doesn't happen to everyone. Some people can have their wisdom teeth removed and never have problems. But for others, improper extraction sites may be ticking time bombs leading to eventual bone loss and resulting tooth loss.

## 11. PROGRESSIVE DENTAL THERAPIES.

**Dentists now have access to tremendous new therapies that can improve your chances of a successful dental procedure and improve your health.** Gone are the days of "Drill it, fill it, and bill it." Factory dentists that still use this philosophy cannot be serving their clients.

### The benefits of using ozone.

**Ozone is one of the key tools in the future of dentistry.** Ozone is great at killing anaerobic bacteria. It can be used as a gas or infused in oil. Ozonated water can also be used to clean out cavitations and extraction sites. Dentists can deliver the ozone gas right into the cavity of a tooth to destroy the bacteria. Then they can fill the cavity after removing the bacteria underneath it. Ozone reduces the number of failed fillings caused by bacteria underneath the filling.[287] Ozone can also be used to clean out the bacteria around root-canal removed teeth and when cleaning out cavitations.

### Vitamin C therapy.

**Vitamin C puts out the fire (oxidative stress) that is being caused by the toxins.** Vitamin C is a substance that can combat toxicity, because it stops the oxidation caused by toxins. An Intravenous (IV) Vitamin C protocol can be administered before, during, and after the procedure, so that the body can detoxify the mercury and other toxins that might get into the body as a result of the procedure. IV Vitamin C helps you to recover from the procedure with as few side effects as possible.

**Vitamin C can be used in many forms.**
- Intravenous Vitamin C can only be obtained under the care of a knowledgeable health practitioner. More and more doctors are becoming aware of the benefits of I.V. Vitamin C for serious problems and are incorporating it into their practices.
- Liposomal Vitamin C is a secondary alternative that allows you to get high blood levels without diarrhea.
- Ascorbate powders are other Vitamin C forms that are cheaper and more readily available. To get as much as possible, gradually take more and more until you get diarrhea (usually around 15 grams a day), then back off a bit. Some people have reported that, when used in a water pik, sodium ascorbate may help to stop or even reverse bone loss.

## Conscious sedation.

**There is a wide margin of safety when a dentist uses conscious sedation.** You can eat the night before, but must be fasting before the procedure.

**Although you are conscious, you won't remember anything.** If the dentist asks you to turn closer or open wider, you will do it, but you won't remember it. If you should need to go to the restroom, a staff member can guide you in there. Much less local anesthetic is needed. You come out of it ten to fifteen minutes after the procedure is finished. In the rare event of an adverse reaction, a reversal drug can be injected into the I.V. Within 30-60 seconds, you will be completely alert and over the effects of the anesthetic.

## Oil pulling.

**Oil pulling is swishing sunflower, sesame or coconut oil around in your mouth for ten or twenty minutes and then spitting it out.** Coconut oil is my favorite, because I like the taste. Coconut oil destroys many harmful kinds of pathogens that are commonly found in the mouth.[288] Oil pulling has been used for centuries as preventative and curative in Ayurvedic (ancient Indian) medicine. Oil pulling purifies the entire system. Good essential oils to use in oil pulling are clove, orange, lemon, grapefruit, bergamot, peppermint, frankincense, and myrrh.

The Ayurvedic texts claim that oil pulling can help over 30 systemic diseases ranging from asthma to migraines to diabetes.[289] Oil pulling removes the fat-soluble bacteria and other toxins in our mouths.[290] [291] It is like using detergent to get the grease out of your clothes and dishes. It has been clinically shown to help with plaque,[292] tooth decay, bad breath,[293] [294] bleeding gums,[295] dry throat, cracked lips,[296] and even strengthening your teeth and jaw. You can put a teaspoon or tablespoon of oil into your mouth first thing in the morning, before you do anything else--before going to the bathroom, taking a shower, or anything. Lightly swish it around for twenty minutes or so. Spit it into the trash, not down the drain, because it will clog the drain. You can put a couple drops of essential oils into the oil. It is recommended to use oil pulling three or four times a week. Doing it more often than that may be too much. Toxic people may get nauseous, because the oil pulling stirs up the toxins. If you get nauseous, you may want to limit the oil pulling to five minutes or less. Less toxic people can handle ten or twenty minutes three or four times a week.

## 12. LEAKY GUT AND ORAL HEALTH.

**If your gut isn't healthy, your mouth can't be healthy.** Leaky gut happens when your intestines become inflamed and stay inflamed over time. Little holes appear in the lining of the intestines when the intestines are inflamed over time. If the condition is allowed to continue, food sensitivities or allergies can develop. Autoimmune disease may also develop.

**No matter what type of wheat is eaten, almost everyone has a problem with it, even if they do not have celiac disease or wheat allergy.** [297] New strains are causing problems in people who previously had no problems with wheat.[298] Many develop irritable bowel syndrome.[299] They may go on to develop auto-immune diseases.[300] Limit the amount of grains consumed, even fermented or sprouted. Sprouted chia or flax seeds help to clean the colon.

**Conventional dairy products may cause leaky gut.** Raw organic, grass-fed, local goat's milk kefir (a cultured dairy drink) could help to heal leaky gut. Kefir is a probiotic food that is the perfect food for your mouth because of the good bacteria it contains. Raw cultured dairy also has plenty of Vitamin D, calcium, and magnesium that help your dental health.

**Excess sugar feeds yeast and certain microorganisms that crowd out good microorganisms.** These pathogenic yeasts can actually eat holes in your gut, causing leaky gut. Sweets should be limited to less than one tablespoon of raw local honey or Manuka honey, which has benefits for the microbiome. Cut way down on fruit.

**Hydrogenated oils like canola and vegetable oils are GMO and are toxic to the gut microbiome.** Replace them with coconut oil, olive oil, flax oil, or ghee. Fish oil that comes from non-mercury-polluted fish is very beneficial in treating inflammation. Krill oil is an exceptional treatment for inflammation.

**Bone broth is the liquid that comes from cartilage, ligaments, and bones after cooking.** The collagen in the bone broth is loaded with amino acids that support us. You can get a collagen powder, or just make your own bone broth.

**Fermented vegetables, like sauerkraut and kimchee, have prebiotics as well as probiotics.** Prebiotics are food for good bacteria and help good bacteria to grow in the gut. These also help your body get to the right pH to heal leaky gut.

**Coconut balances out candida and yeast, because coconut products are anti-microbial.** Use all forms of coconut liberally in your diet.

**Vitamin D supports the good anti-microbials** (which target the bad bacteria), so that you can keep a good balance of bacteria in the microbiome, in the mouth, as well as the gut. If you are deficient in Vitamin D, you will have weaker bones and teeth and more fragile jawbones. Indoor jobs and inappropriate fear of sunlight have reduced the blood levels of Vitamin D in modern cultures to dangerously low levels. You may not have enough bone growth to fit all the teeth into your mouth, crowding out the wisdom teeth.

**Relax while you eat.** Chew each bite into liquid, so that the enzymes in your saliva break down your food. If you are deficient in acid in your stomach, chewing thoroughly greatly decreases the problems from low hydrochloric acid. Inadequate stomach acid produces putrefaction of food in the small intestine.

**Get away from toxins, eat better, and sleep better.** Prescription antibiotics kill off the good bacteria and make it much more likely that we will need antibiotics in the future.

**Take a good probiotic.** Unfortunately, most of the probiotics on the market are very poor. Get your probiotics from the refrigerator in the health food store. Look for one with the greatest number of different strains.

**It is best to get your probiotics from food.** Some experts believe that probiotics are killed 100% by the stomach acid. Other experts believe that some probiotic gets through to the small intestine, but all agree that probiotic foods get through to the small intestine.

**Look for soil-based organisms,** probiotics that we get from the soil. Most of us do not get enough soil-based organisms, because we are not getting dirty from sleeping on the ground and because we eat food that has been thoroughly washed. Two important soil-based probiotics are Bacillus Subtilus and Lactobacillus Plantarum.

**Digestive enzymes may also be very helpful** to those with digestive problems, because they help to break down the food you are eating.

**L-glutamine is another very helpful supplement to those with digestive issues.** It is an amino acid that helps to protect the gut lining.

**Exercise can also help with leaky gut.** Exercise helps to get your mind off your problems. Emotional stress can be just as damaging to our health as a bad diet. Exercise increases circulation, reduces inflammation, and balances stress hormones. Over exercising is just another bad stress. Exercise daily and moderately.

## 13. HEAL WITH ESSENTIAL OILS.

**There is no standardization or regulation of essential oils.** You have to try them out and see for yourself if you get results.

**Never use essential oils undiluted, or in your eyes or mucus membranes.** Do not take internally unless working with a qualified and expert practitioner. Keep away from children. When applying an essential oil to your skin, dilute the oil in an appropriate carrier and do a small patch test to an insensitive part of the body. Some oils should be avoided while pregnant and in liver and kidney conditions. Good essential oils to use before oral surgery to reduce pain and anxiety are lavender, orange, or chamomile.

### Essential oils to use in specific conditions.

**Abscess.**
Clove, helichrysum, frankincense, roman chamomile, tea tree

**Bad Breath (Halitosis).**
Peppermint, lavender, patchouli

**Cavities.**
Tea tree oil, peppermint, eucalyptus

**Gums.**
Lavender, myrrh, tea tree oil, helichrysum, roman chamomile

**Gum Disease/Gingivitis.**
Myrrh, tea tree, helichrysum, rose

**Mouth Ulcers.**
Basil, orange, myrrh

**Teething Pain.**
Lavender, clove, chamomile

**Toothache.**
Clove, tea Tree Oil

### Specific essential oils for oral health:

**Bergamot.**
Bergamot can be applied on infected teeth or used as a mouthwash to kill oral germs and protect teeth from the development of cavities.

**Cajuput.**
Enhances tissue healing of shrinking gums/pyorrhea.

### Chamomile.
Enhances tissue healing.

### Cinnamon.
Cinnamon essential oil has the greatest antimicrobial potency against streptococcus mutans, the bacteria responsible for tooth decay.[301]

### Clove.
Use for sensitive teeth, gingivitis, bleeding gums, canker sores. Clove essential oil has been used in traditional Chinese medicine for hundreds of years to relieve tooth pain. Clove oil acts as a powerful disinfectant and local anesthetic. Clinical research demonstrated that clove inhibits many pathogenic bacteria.

### Cypress.
For bleeding gums.

### Eucalyptus.
Mix the medicinal-grade oil with grapeseed or almond oil and massage gums affected by periodontal disease.

### Lavender.
Lavender enhances blood circulation and tissue formation and smells great! Use for blood blisters and canker sores. You can try it straight, or for people with sensitive skin, dilute with fractionated coconut oil, so there is no burning.

### Lemon.
Enhances gum tissue healing.

### Myrrh.
Myrrh supports gum health and heals mouth ulcers. May also assist gum tissue health by supporting the flow of blood to the tissue.

### Peppermint.
Very effective at killing anaerobic bacteria.

### Rosemary.
Rosemary has antimicrobial activity against numerous bacteria, yeasts and fungi and increases circulation.

### Spearmint.
A strong antiseptic.

### Tea tree.
Pain killer and kills infective microorganisms.

### Thyme.
Antimicrobial and antibacterial activity.

## 14. CONCLUSION.

We sincerely hope that this book has opened your eyes to the limitations of conventional dentistry and the advantages of cleaning up the problems in your mouth by seeing a biological dentist and getting a total dental revision. After reading this book, you should now understand how dental issues can lead to the development of a wide array of disease processes. You should also now see how most dentists, conforming to the standard of care mandated by their state's dental boards, perform procedures that may harm your health.

**These harmful procedures include the introduction of toxic metals and other toxic chemicals into your mouth.** These toxic materials will continue to poison your body until you have them removed. At that point, you must work hard for the rest of your life to detoxify them. You can never completely get them out, but, as time goes by and you continue your detoxification efforts, you can lower their concentration, and your health should improve.

**In addition to putting toxic materials into your mouth, another extremely harmful treatment performed by conventional dentists is the root canal procedure.** As the immune system tries to cope with the bacterial infection caused by the root canal procedure, untold suffering results.

**The faulty extraction techniques of conventional dentistry may also lead to further dental and other health problems.** These faulty extraction techniques lead to the development of infections and cavitations, or holes in the jawbones. These cavitations spread throughout the jawbones, loosening teeth and seeding infection throughout the body.

**Now that you have learned about the negative consequences of conventional dentistry, it is time for you to take action.** Begin cleaning up the problems in your mouth using the techniques of careful brushing, irrigation, flossing, using essential oils, and application of ozonated olive oil.

**Begin researching biological dentists.** If you cannot find one in your area, do not hesitate to travel to the office of a good biological dentist, even if it costs more than seeing a dentist in your own area. After all, what is your health worth? To learn more about the Hal Huggins protocol and to find a dentist who has been certified in Huggins' methodology, go to http://hugginsappliedhealing.com or call 1-866-948-4638, or E-mail: kim@drhuggins.com. Thanks for reading our books and good luck on your journey toward vibrantly fantastic health!

# REFERENCES.

[1] Reinhardt JW. Side-effects: mercury contribution to body burden from dental amalgam. *Adv Dent Res.* 1992 Sep;6:110-3. Review.

[2] Thornton-Evans G, Eke P, Wei L, Palmer A, Moeti R, Hutchins S, Borrell LN; Centers for Disease Control and Prevention (CDC). Periodontitis among adults aged≥30 years - United States, 2009-2010. *MMWR Surveill Summ.* 2013 Nov 22;62 Suppl3:129-35.

[3] Lechner J, von Baehr V. RANTES and fibroblast growth factor 2 in jawbone cavitations: triggers for systemic disease? *Int J Gen Med.* 2013 Apr 22;6:277-90.

[4] Brotóns A, Peñarrocha M. Orofacial neurogenic pain and maxillofacial ischemic osteonecrosis. A review. *Med Oral.* 2003 May-Jul;8(3):157-65.

[5] Moorer WR, Thoden van Velzen SK, Wesselink PR. Abscess formation induced in rabbits with bacteria-filled subcutaneous implants that simulate the infected dental root canal. *Oral Surg Oral Med Oral Pathol.* 1985 Jun;59(6):642-6.

[6] Breebaart AC, Bijlsma JW, van Eden W. 16-year remission of rheumatoid arthritis after unusually vigorous treatment of closed dental foci. *Clin Exp Rheumatol.* 2002 Jul-Aug;20(4):555-7.

[7] Pasqualini D, Bergandi L, Palumbo L, Borraccino A, Dambra V, Alovisi M, Migliaretti G, Ferraro G, Ghigo D, Bergerone S, Scotti N, Aimetti M, Berutti E.Association among oral health, apical periodontitis, CD14 polymorphisms, and coronary heart disease in middle-aged adults. *J Endod.* 2012 Dec;38(12):1570-7.

[8] Ebersole JL, Graves CL, Gonzalez OA, Dawson D 3rd, Morford LA, Huja PE, Hartsfield JK Jr, Huja SS, Pandruvada S, Wallet SM. Aging, inflammation, immunity and periodontal disease. *Periodontol 2000.* 2016 Oct;72(1):54-75.

[9] Liljestrand JM, Mäntylä P, Paju S, Buhlin K, Kopra KA, Persson GR, HernandezM, Nieminen MS, Sinisalo J, Tjäderhane L, Pussinen PJ. Association of Endodontic Lesions with Coronary Artery Disease. *J Dent Res.* 2016 Jul 27.

[10] Mahendra J, Mahendra L, Kurian VM, Jaishankar K, Mythilli R. 16S rRNA-based detection of oral pathogens in coronary atherosclerotic plaque. *Indian J Dent Res.* 2010 Apr-Jun;21(2):248-52.

[11] Fitzpatrick SG, Katz J. The association between periodontal disease and cancer: a review of the literature. *J Dent.* 2010 Feb;38(2):83-95.

[12] Badran Z, Struillou X, Verner C, Clee T, Rakic M, Martinez MC, Soueidan A. Periodontitis as a risk factor for systemic disease: Are microparticles the missing link? *Med Hypotheses.* 2015 Jun;84(6):555-6.

[13] Adams WR, Spolnik KJ, Bouquot JE. Maxillofacial osteonecrosis in a patient with multiple "idiopathic" facial pains. *J Oral Pathol Med.* 1999 Oct;28(9):423-32.

[14] Echeverria D, Aposhian HV, Woods JS, Heyer NJ, Aposhian MM, Bittner AC Jr,Mahurin RK, Cianciola M. Neurobehavioral effects from exposure to dental amalgam Hg(o): new distinctions between recent exposure and Hg body burden. *FASEB J.* 1998 Aug;12(11):971-80.

[15] Chaari N, Chebel S, Merchaoui I, Kerkeni A, Neffati F, Najjar F, Akrout M. Neuropsychological Effects of Mercury Exposure Among Dentists in Monastir City. *Recent Pat Inflamm Allergy Drug Discov.* 2015;9(2):151-8.

[16] Hawton K, Agerbo E, Simkin S, Platt B, Mellanby RJ. Risk of suicide in medical and related occupational groups: a national study based on Danish case population-based registers. *J Affect Disord.* 2011 Nov;134(1-3):320-6.

[17] Murtomaa H. Work-related complaints of dentists and dental assistants. *Int Arch Occup Environ Health.* 1982;50(3):231-6.

[18] Hashim R, Al-Ali K. Health of dentists in United Arab Emirates. *Int Dent J.* 2013 Feb;63(1):26-9.

[19] Colson DG. A safe protocol for amalgam removal. *J Environ Public Health.* 2012;2012:517391.

[20] http://iaomt.org

[21] http://paracelsus.ch/dentistry-and-biological-medicine/?lang=en

[22] Wright YL, Swartz JM. *Bioidentical Hormones Made Easy*. Lulu Press. 2011.
[23] Kern JK, Geier DA, Bjørklund G, King PG, Homme KG, Haley BE, Sykes LK, Geier MR. Evidence supporting a link between dental amalgams and chronic illness, fatigue, depression, anxiety, and suicide. *Neuro Endocrinol Lett.2014;35(7):537-52. Review.*
[24] Siblerud RL, Kienholz E. Evidence that mercury from silver dental fillings may be an etiological factor in multiple sclerosis. *Sci Total Environ. 1994 Mar15;142(3):191-205.*
[25] Huggins HA, Levy TE. Cerebrospinal fluid protein changes in multiple sclerosis after dental amalgam removal. *Altern Med Rev. 1998 Aug;3(4):295-300.*
[26] Huggins HA. Proposed role of dental amalgam toxicity in leukemia and hematopoietic dyscrasias. *International Journal of Biosocial and Medical Research. 1989. 11:84-93.*
[27] Echeverria D, Woods JS, Heyer NJ, Rohlman DS, Farin FM, Bittner AC Jr, Li T, Garabedian C. Chronic low-level mercury exposure, BDNF polymorphism, and associations with cognitive and motor function. *Neurotoxicol Teratol. 2005 Nov-Dec;27(6):781-96.*
[28] Lechner J, von Baehr V. RANTES and fibroblast growth factor 2 in jawbone cavitations: triggers for systemic disease? *Int J Gen Med. 2013 Apr 22;6:277-90.*
[29] Zanella SG, Roberti di Sarsina P. Personalization of multiple sclerosis treatments: using the chelation therapy approach. *Explore (NY). 2013 Jul-Aug;9(4):244-8.*
[30] Via CS, Nguyen P, Niculescu F, Papadimitriou J, Hoover D, Silbergeld EK. Low-dose exposure to inorganic mercury accelerates disease and mortality in acquired murine lupus. *Environ Health Perspect. 2003 Aug;111(10):1273-7.*
[31] Leech MT, Bartold PM. The association between rheumatoid arthritis and periodontitis. *Best Pract Res Clin Rheumatol. 2015 Apr;29(2):189-201.*
[32] **Furuya T, Maeda S, Momohara S, Taniguchi A, Yamanaka H. Dental treatments, tooth extractions, and osteonecrosis of the jaw in Japanese patients with rheumatoid arthritis: results from the IORRA cohort study.** *J Bone Miner Metab. 2016 Jul 2.*
[33] Carocci A, Rovito N, Sinicropi MS, Genchi G. Mercury toxicity and neurodegenerative effects. *Rev Environ Contam Toxicol. 2014;229:1-18.*
[34] Chin-Chan M, Navarro-Yepes J, Quintanilla-Vega B. Environmental pollutants as risk factors for neurodegenerative disorders: Alzheimer and Parkinson diseases. *Front Cell Neurosci. 2015 Apr 10;9:124.*
[35] Pendergrass JC, Haley BE, Vimy MJ, Winfield SA, Lorscheider FL. Mercury vapor inhalation inhibits binding of GTP to tubulin in rat brain: similarity to a molecular lesion in Alzheimer diseased brain. *Neurotoxicology. 1997;18(2):315-24.*
[36] Louhelainen AM, Aho J, Tuomisto S, Aittoniemi J, Vuento R, Karhunen PJ, Pessi T. Oral bacterial DNA findings in pericardial fluid. *J Oral Microbiol. 2014 Nov 19;6:25835.*
[37] Ryder MI, Nittayananta W, Coogan M, Greenspan D, Greenspan JS. Periodontal disease in HIV/AIDS. *Periodontol 2000. 2012 Oct;60(1):78-97.*
[38] Novotna M, Podzimek S, Broukal Z, Lencova E, Duskova J. Periodontal Diseases and Dental Caries in Children with Type 1 Diabetes Mellitus. *Mediators Inflamm. Epub 2015 Aug 4. Review.*
[39] Basha S, Shivalinga Swamy H, Noor Mohamed R. Maternal Periodontitis as a Possible Risk Factor for Preterm Birth and Low Birth Weight--A Prospective Study. *Oral Health Prev Dent. 2015;13(6):537-44.*
[40] Tavares M, Lindefjeld Calabi KA, San Martin L. Systemic diseases and oral health. *Dent Clin North Am. 2014 Oct;58(4):797-814.*
[41] Pyysalo MJ, Pyysalo LM, Pessi T, Karhunen PJ, Lehtimäki T, Oksala N, Öhman JE. Bacterial DNA findings in ruptured and unruptured intracranial aneurysms. *ActaOdontol Scand. 2016;74(4):315-20.*
[42] Pyysalo MJ, Pyysalo LM, Pessi T, Karhunen PJ, Öhman JE. The connection between ruptured cerebral aneurysms and odontogenic bacteria. *J Neurol Neurosurg Psychiatry. 2013 Nov;84(11):1214-8.*
[43] Weaver T, Auclair PL, Taybos GM. An amalgam tattoo causing local and systemic disease? *Oral Surg*

*Oral Med Oral Pathol. 1987 Jan;63(1):137-40.*
[44] http://www.issels.com/treatment-summary/
[45] Issels J. [Results and insights subsequent to four year clinico-internal therapy of incurable cancer]. *Hippokrates. 1954 Aug 31;25(16):514-29.* German.
[46] Issels, J. *Cancer: A Second Opinion.* Square One Publishers, Inc. Garden City Park, NY. 2005.
[47] Vartazarian ND. [Palatal tonsil changes and interstitial microbial foci in chronic tonsillitis]. *Arkh Patol. 1981;43(5):10-5.* Russian.
[48] Misiukiewicz K, Posner M. Role of Prophylactic Bilateral Tonsillectomy as a Cancer Preventive Strategy. *Cancer Prev Res (Phila). 2015 Jul;8(7):580-2.*
[49] Rose NR. Prediction and Prevention of Autoimmune Disease in the 21st Century: A Review and Preview. *Am J Epidemiol. 2016 Mar 1;183(5):403-6.*
[50] http://www.aarda.org/autoimmune-information/autoimmune-statistics/
[51] Ji J, Sundquist J, Sundquist K. Gender-specific incidence of autoimmune diseases from national registers. *J Autoimmun. 2016 May;69:102-6.*
[52] Meyers A. *The Autoimmune Solution: Prevent and Reverse the Full Spectrum of Inflammatory Symptoms and Diseases.* Harper Collins. New York, N.Y. 2015.
[53] Nielsen PR, Kragstrup TW, Deleuran BW, Benros ME. Infections as risk factor for autoimmune diseases - A nationwide study. *J Autoimmun. 2016 Jun 4.*
[54] Newman MG. Anaerobic oral and dental infection. *Rev Infect Dis. 1984 Mar-Apr;6 Suppl 1:S107-14.* Review.
[55] Lerner A, Matthias T. Changes in intestinal tight junction permeability associated with industrial food additives explain the rising incidence of autoimmune disease. *Autoimmun Rev. 2015 Jun;14(6):479-89.*
[56] Mutter J. Is dental amalgam safe for humans? The opinion of the scientific committee of the European Commission. *J Occup Med Toxicol. 2011 Jan 13;6(1):2.*
[57] Hultman P, Lindh U, Hörsted-Bindslev P. Activation of the immune system and systemic immune-complex deposits in Brown Norway rats with dental amalgam restorations. *J Dent Res. 1998 Jun;77(6):1415-25.*
[58] Porcelli B, Pozza A, Bizzaro N, Fagiolini A, Costantini MC, Terzuoli L,Ferretti F. Association between stressful life events and autoimmune diseases: A systematic review and meta-analysis of retrospective case-control studies. *Autoimmun Rev. 2016 Apr;15(4):325-34.*
[59] Louhelainen AM, Aho J, Tuomisto S, Aittoniemi J, Vuento R, Karhunen PJ, Pessi T. Oral bacterial DNA findings in pericardial fluid. *J Oral Microbiol. 2014 Nov19;6:25835.*
[60] T.E.R.F.New DNA study confirms decades old research that root canals contain toxic bacterium that may be the 'root' cause of many diseases. *Root Canal News Release.*
[61] Miettinen H, Lehto S, Saikku P, Haffner SM, Rönnemaa T, Pyörälä K, Laakso M. Association of Chlamydia pneumoniae and acute coronary heart disease events in non-insulin dependent diabetic and non-diabetic subjects in Finland. *Eur Heart J. 1996 May;17(5):682-8.*
[62] Ziebolz D, Rost C, Schmidt J, Waldmann-Beushausen R, Schöndube FA, Mausberg RF, Danner BC. Periodontal Bacterial DNA and Their Link to Human Cardiac Tissue: Findings of a Pilot Study. *Thorac Cardiovasc Surg. 2015 Oct 5.*
[63] Oliveira FA, Forte CP, Silva PG, Lopes CB, Montenegro RC, Santos ÂK, Sobrinho CR, Mota MR, Sousa FB, Alves AP. Molecular Analysis of Oral Bacteria in Heart Valve of Patients With Cardiovascular Disease by Real-Time Polymerase Chain Reaction. *Medicine (Baltimore). 2015 Nov;94(47):e2067.*
[64] Hosomi N, Aoki S, Matsuo K, Deguchi K, Masugata H, Murao K, Ichihara N, OhyamaH, Dobashi H, Nezu T, Ohtsuki T, Yasuda O, Soejima H, Ogawa H, Izumi Y, Kohno M, Tanaka J, Matsumoto M. Association of serum antiperiodontal pathogen antibody with ischemic stroke. *Cerebrovasc Dis. 2012;34(5-6):385-92.*
[65] Valachovic R, Hargreaves JA. Dental implications of brain abscess in children with congenital heart disease. Case report and review of the literature. *OralSurg Oral Med Oral Pathol. 1979 Dec;48(6):495-*

500.

[66] Shanker J, Setty P, Arvind P, Nair J, Bhasker D, Balakrishna G, Kakkar VV. Relationship between periodontal disease, Porphyromonas gingivalis, peripheral vascular resistance markers and coronary artery disease in Asian Indians. *Thromb Res.* 2013 Jul;132(1):e8-14.

[67] Elkaïm R, Dahan M, Kocgozlu L, Werner S, Kanter D, Kretz JG, Tenenbaum H. Prevalence of periodontal pathogens in subgingival lesions, atherosclerotic plaques and healthy blood vessels: a preliminary study. *J Periodontal Res.* 2008 Apr;43(2):224-31.

[68] Bouquot JE, LaMarche MG: Ischemic Osteonecrosis under fixed partial denture pontics: Radiographic and microscopic features in 38 patients with chronic pain. *J Prosthetic Dent* 81: 148-158.

[69] Castoldi AF, Coccini T, Ceccatelli S, Manzo L. Neurotoxicity and molecular effects of methylmercury. *Brain Res Bull.* 2001 May 15;55(2):197-203. Review.

[70] Powell JJ, Van de Water J, Gershwin ME. Evidence for the role of environmental agents in the initiation or progression of autoimmune conditions. *Environ Health Perspect.* 1999 Oct;107 Suppl 5:667-72. Review.

[71] Gall H. [Allergies to dental materials and dental pharmacologic agents]. *Hautarzt.* 1983 Jul;34(7):326-31. German.

[72] Marchi A, Piana G. [Amalgam and the toxicological risks of mercury. A review of the argument]. *Minerva Stomatol.* 1995 Jun;44(6):311-8. Review. Italian.

[73] Breebaart AC, Bijlsma JW, van Eden W. 16-year remission of rheumatoid arthritis after unusually vigorous treatment of closed dental foci. *Clin Exp Rheumatol.* 2002 Jul-Aug;20(4):555-7.

[74] Koch F, Breil P, Marroquín BB, Gawehn J, Kunkel M. Abscess of the orbit arising 48 h after root canal treatment of a maxillary first molar. *Int Endod J.* 2006 Aug;39(8):657-64.

[75] van der Meulen TA, Harmsen HJ, Bootsma H, Spijkervet FK, Kroese FG, Vissink A. The microbiome systemic diseases connection. *Oral Dis.* 2016 Mar 8.

[76] Diamanti AP, Manuela Rosado M, Laganà B, D'Amelio R. Microbiota and chronic inflammatory arthritis: an interwoven link. *J Transl Med.* 2016 Aug 4;14(1):233.

[77] http://iaomt.org/find-a-doctor/questions-for-your-dentist/

[78] Gabrio T, Benedikt G, Broser S, Felder-Kennel A, Fichtner G, Horras-Hun G, Jovanovic S, Kirsch H, Kouros B, Link B, Maisner V, Piechotowski I, Rzonca E, Schick KH, Schrimpf M, Schröder S, Schwenk M, Spöker-Maas K, Weidner U, Wuthe J, Zöllner I. [10 years of observation by public health offices in Baden-Württemberg--assessment of human biomonitoring for mercury due to dental amalgam fillings and other sources]. *Gesundheitswesen.* 2003 May;65(5):327-35.German.

[79] Lorscheider FL, Vimy MJ, Summers AO. Mercury exposure from "silver" tooth fillings: emerging evidence questions a traditional dental paradigm. *FASEB J.*1995 Apr;9(7):504-8. Review.

[80] http://mercurymadness.info/videos/

[81] http://www.prnewswire.com/news-releases/who-lauded-for-supporting-amalgam-phase-down-ban-on-mercury-in-skin-cosmetics-as-treaty-negotiations-start-in-stockholm-96160449.html

[82] Mutter J, Naumann J, Walach H, Daschner F. [Amalgam risk assessment with coverage of references up to 2005]. *Gesundheitswesen.* 2005 Mar;67(3):204-16. Review. German.

[83] Bensefa-Colas L, Andujar P, Descatha A. [Mercury poisoning]. *Rev Med Interne.* 2011 Jul;32(7):416-24. Review. French.

[84] Nordberg GF. Current concepts in the assessment of effects of metals in chronic low-level exposures--considerations of experimental and epidemiological evidence. *Sci Total Environ.* 1988 Jun 1;71(3):243-52. Review.

[85] Sandborgh-Englund G, Elinder CG, Johanson G, Lind B, Skare I, Ekstrand J. The absorption, blood levels, and excretion of mercury after a single dose of mercury vapor in humans. *Toxicol Appl Pharmacol.* 1998 May;150(1):146-53.

[86] Chew CL, Soh G, Lee AS, Yeoh TS. Long-term dissolution of mercury from a non-mercury-releasing

amalgam. *Clin Prev Dent. 1991 May-Jun;13(3):5-7.*
[87] Svare CW, Peterson LC, Reinhardt JW, Boyer DB, Frank CW, Gay DD, Cox RD. The effect of dental amalgams on mercury levels in expired air. *J Dent Res. 1981 Sep;60(9):1668-71.*
[88] Guzzi G, Grandi M, Cattaneo C, Calza S, Minoia C, Ronchi A, Gatti A, Severi G. Dental amalgam and mercury levels in autopsy tissues: food for thought. *Am J Forensic Med Pathol. 2006 Mar;27(1):42-5.*
[89] Geier DA, Carmody T, Kern JK, King PG, Geier MR. A significant dose-dependent relationship between mercury exposure from dental amalgams and kidney integrity biomarkers: a further assessment of the Casa Pia children's dental amalgam trial. *Hum Exp Toxicol. 2013 Apr;32(4):434-40.*
[90] Nylander M, Friberg L, Lind B. Mercury concentrations in the human brain and kidneys in relation to exposure from dental amalgam fillings. *Swed Dent J.1987;11(5):179-87.*
[91] T.E.R.F. New evidence correlates chronic fatigue with common dental materials. *T.E.R.F .D-Day Media Ch Fatigue.*
[92] Kern JK, Geier DA, Bjørklund G, King PG, Homme KG, Haley BE, Sykes LK, Geier MR. Evidence supporting a link between dental amalgams and chronic illness, fatigue, depression, anxiety, and suicide. *Neuro Endocrinol Lett.2014;35(7):537-52. Review.*
[93] Cordier S, Deplan F, Mandereau L, Hemon D. Paternal exposure to mercury and spontaneous abortions. *Br J Ind Med. 1991 Jun;48(6):375-81.*
[94] Chang LW, Wade PR, Pounds JG, Reuhl KR. Prenatal and neonatal toxicology and pathology of heavy metals. *Adv Pharmacol Chemother. 1980;17:195-231. Review.*
[95] Marsh DO, Clarkson TW, Cox C, Myers GJ, Amin-Zaki L, Al-Tikriti S. Fetal methylmercury poisoning. Relationship between concentration in single strands of maternal hair and child effects. *Arch Neurol. 1987 Oct;44(10):1017-22.*
[96] Wataha JC, Craig RG, Hanks CT. The release of elements of dental casting alloys into cell-culture medium. *J Dent Res. 1991 Jun;70(6):1014-8.*
[97] Friberg, Lars, Nordberg, Gunnar F. and Vouk, Velimir B. (eds.), Handbook on the Toxicology of Metals, Vol. I. Elsesvier Science Publishing Co., New York, NY,1986.
[98] Ganser AL, Kirschner DA. The interaction of mercurials with myelin: comparison of in vitro and in vivo effects. *Neurotoxicology. 1985 Spring;6(1):63-77.*
[99] Henriksson J, Tjälve H. Uptake of inorganic mercury in the olfactory bulbs via olfactory pathways in rats. *Environ Res. 1998 May;77(2):130-40.*
[100] Sjöstrand J. Fast and slow components of axoplasmic transport in the hypoglossal and vagus nerves of the rabbit. *Brain Res. 1970 Mar 17;18(3):461-7.*
[101] Huggins, H.A. *It's all in your head. The link between mercury amalgams and illness.* Hal A. Huggins, D.D.S., M.S. 1993.
[102] Burger WG, van den Heuvel J, Kolsteeg E, Schuurs AH. [Amalgam use and mercury emission in the Netherlands]. *Ned Tijdschr Tandheelkd. 1997 Mar;104(3):95-8. Review. Dutch.*
[103] Yoshida M, Kishimoto T, Yamamura Y, Tabuse M, Akama Y, Satoh H. [Amount of mercury from dental amalgam filling released into the atmosphere by cremation]. *Nihon Koshu Eisei Zasshi. 1994 Jul;41(7):618-24. Japanese.*
[104] Noguchi K, Shimizu M, Moriwaki K, Jinnouchi K, Sairenji E. [Activation analysis of mercury in head hair of dentists (author's transl)]. *Radioisotopes. 1980 May;29(5):221-6. Japanese.*
[105] Mumtaz R, Ali Khan A, Noor N, Humayun S. Amalgam use and waste management by Pakistani dentists: an environmental perspective. *East Mediterr Health J. 2010 Mar;16(3):334-9.*
[106] Khwaja MA, Abbasi MS. Mercury poisoning dentistry: high-level indoor air mercury contamination at selected dental sites. *Rev Environ Health. 2014;29(1-2):29-31.*
[107] Hilt B, Svendsen K, Syversen T, Aas O, Qvenild T, Sletvold H, Melø I. Occurrence of cognitive symptoms in dental assistants with previous occupational exposure to metallic mercury. *Neurotoxicology. 2009 Nov;30(6):1202-6*
[108] Jones L, Bunnell J, Stillman J. A 30-year follow-up of residual effects on New Zealand School Dental

Nurses, from occupational mercury exposure. *Hum Exp Toxicol. 2007 Apr;26(4):367-74.*
[109] Sancho FM, Ruiz CN. Risk of suicide amongst dentists: myth or reality? *Int Dent J. 2010 Dec;60(6):411-8. Review.*
[110] Schiønning JD, Poulsen EH, Møller-Madsen B, Danscher G. Ultrastructural localization of mercury in rat dorsal root ganglia after exposure to mercury vapor. *Prog Histochem Cytochem. 1991;23(1-4):249-55.*
[111] Bergfors E, Hermansson G, Nyström Kronander U, Falk L, Valter L, Trollfors B. How common are long-lasting, intensely itching vaccination granulomas and contact allergy to aluminium induced by currently used pediatric vaccines? A prospective cohort study. *Eur J Pediatr. 2014 Oct;173(10):1297-307.*
[112] Soldin OP, O'Mara DM, Aschner M. Thyroid hormones and methylmercury toxicity. *Biol Trace Elem Res. 2008 Winter;126(1-3):1-12.*
[113] Chen A, Kim SS, Chung E, Dietrich KN. Thyroid hormones in relation to lead, mercury, and cadmium exposure in the National Health and Nutrition Examination Survey, 2007-2008. *Environ Health Perspect. 201 Feb;121(2):181-6.*
[114] Gallagher CM, Meliker JR. Mercury and thyroid autoantibodies in U.S. women. *NHANES 2007-2008. Environ Int. 2012 Apr;40:39-43.*
[115] Jarvis group. Collected correspondence between D.C. Jarvis and numerous letter writers. Information collected and evaluated between 1920 and 1950 by Jarvis, who disseminated findings to group.
[116] Homme KG, Kern JK, Haley BE, Geier DA, King PG, Sykes LK, Geier MR. New science challenges old notion that mercury dental amalgam is safe. *Biometals. 2014 Feb;27(1):19-24. Review.*
[117] Pleva J. Mercury from dental amalgams: exposure and effects. *Int J Risk Saf Med. 1992;3(1):1-22.*
[118] Bautista LE, Stein JH, Morgan BJ, Stanton N, Young T, Nieto FJ. Association of blood and hair mercury with blood pressure and vascular reactivity. *WMJ. 2009 Aug;108(5):250-2.*
[119] Liu XL, Wang HB, Sun CW, Xiong XS, Chen Z, Li ZS, Han B, Yang G. [The clinical analysis of mercury poisoning in 92 cases]. *Zhonghua Nei Ke Za Zhi. 2011 Aug;50(8):687-9. Chinese.*
[120] Goldberg RL, Kaplan SR, Fuller GC. Effect of heavy metals on human rheumatoid synovial cell proliferation and collagen synthesis. *Biochem Pharmacol. 1983 Sep15;32(18):2763-6.*
[121] Bigazzi PE. Autoimmunity and heavy metals. *Lupus. 1994 Dec;3(6):449-53. Review.*
[122] Siblerud RL. A comparison of mental health of multiple sclerosis patients with silver/mercury dental fillings and those with fillings removed. *Psychol Rep. 1992 Jun;70(3 Pt 2):1139-51.*
[123] Ingalls TH. Epidemiology, etiology, and prevention of multiple sclerosis. Hypothesis and fact. *Am J Forensic Med Pathol. 1983 Mar;4(1):55-61.*
[124] Mano Y, Takayanagi T, Abe T, Takizawa Y. [Amyotrophic lateral sclerosis and mercury--preliminary report]. *Rinsho Shinkeigaku. 1990 Nov;30(11):1275-7. Japanese.*
[125] Hybenova M, Hrda P, Procházková J, Stejskal V, Sterzl I. The role of environmental factors in autoimmune thyroiditis. *Neuro Endocrinol Lett. 2010;31(3):283-9. Review.*
[126] Yoshida S, Gershwin ME. Autoimmunity and selected environmental factors of disease induction. *Semin Arthritis Rheum. 1993 Jun;22(6):399-419. Review.*
[127] Zheng Y, Monestier M. Inhibitory signal override increases susceptibility to mercury-induced autoimmunity. *J Immunol. 2003 Aug 1;171(3):1596-601.*
[128] Wang L, Wang FS, Gershwin ME. Human autoimmune diseases: a comprehensive update. *J Intern Med. 2015 Oct;278(4):369-95.*
[129] Rothwell JA, Boyd PJ. Amalgam dental fillings and hearing loss. *Int J Audiol. 2008 Dec;47(12):770-6.*
[130] Huggins, H.A. *It's all in your head. The link between mercury amalgams and illness.* Hal A. Huggins, D.D.S., M.S. 1993. p. 6-7.
[131] New red blood cell bio "marker" test provides key to understanding dental toxicity and disease. *T.E.R.F. Red Blood Cells News Release (1.0).*

[132] Bouquot JE: Characterization and identification of chemical toxicants isolated from cavitational material and infected root canalled teeth; in situ testing of teeth for toxicity and infection. *Proceedings of Annual Meeting, International Academy of Oral Medicine and Toxicology; San Diego, CA; 1997.*

[133] Lechner J, von Baehr V. Rantes and fibroblast growth factor in jawbone cavitations; Triggers for systemic disease? *International Journal of Medicine 2013: 6, 277-290.*

[134] Lechner J. Chronic osteonecrosis of jawbone (NICO): Unknown trigger for systemic disease and a possible new integrative approach? *J Altern Med Res 2013;5(3):243-250.*

[135] Lechner J., von Baehr V. Hyperactive signaling pathways of chemokine RANTES/CCL5 in osteopathies of jawbone in breast cancer patients—case report and research. *Breast Cancer: Basic and Clinical Research 2014: 8, 89-96.*

[136] Huggins, H.A. It's all in your head. The link between mercury amalgams and illness. Hal A. Huggins, D.D.S., M.S. 1993.

[137] Schuurs AH, van Amerongen JP. [Amalgam. VIII. Substitute for amalgam: the biocompatibility of composite restorations]. *Ned Tijdschr Tandheelkd. 1993 Sep;100(9):389-91.* Dutch.

[138] Clifford Consulting and Research. Should I be worried about aluminum in fillings and crowns? Colorado Springs, CO. 2008

[139] http://www.dentalconfessions.com/

[140] Hoover R. et al (1991). Fluoridation of Drinking Water and Subsequent Cancer Incidence and Mortality. In Review of Fluoride: Benefits and Risks, Report of the Ad Hoc Committee on Fluoride of the Committee to Coordinate Environmental Health and Related Programs. *US Public Health Service, pp E1-E51.*

[141] Yiamouyiannis (1993). Fluoridation and Cancer. The Biology and Epidemiology of Bone and Oral Cancer Related to Fluoridation. *Fluoride, 26, 83-96.*

[142] Smith GE. The action of fluoride in teeth and bone. *Med Hypotheses. 1986 Feb;19(2):139-54.*

[143] Lütfioğlu M, Sakallıoğlu EE, Sakallıoğlu U, Gülbahar MY, Muğlalı M, Baş B, Aksoy A. Excessive fluoride intake alters the MMP-2, TIMP-1 and TGF-β levels of periodontal soft tissues: an experimental study in rabbits. *Clin Oral Investig. 2012 Dec;16(6):1563-70.*

[144] Valdez-Jiménez L, Soria Fregozo C, Miranda Beltrán ML, Gutiérrez Coronado O, Pérez Vega MI. Effects of the fluoride on the central nervous system. *Neurologia. 2011 Jun;26(5):297-300.*

[145] Valdez-Jiménez L, Soria Fregozo C, Miranda Beltrán ML, Gutiérrez Coronado O, Pérez Vega MI. Effects of the fluoride on the central nervous system. *Neurologia. 2011 Jun;26(5):297-300.*

[146] Choi AL, Zhang Y, Sun G, Bellinger DC, Wang K, Yang XJ, Li JS, Zheng Q, Fu Y, Grandjean P. Association of lifetime exposure to fluoride and cognitive functions in Chinese children: a pilot study. *Neurotoxicol Teratol. 2015 Jan-Feb;47:96-101.*

[147] Das K, Mondal NK. Dental fluorosis and urinary fluoride concentration as a reflection of fluoride exposure and its impact on IQ level and BMI of children of Laxmisagar, Simlapal Block of Bankura District, W.B., India. *Environ Monit Assess. 2016 Apr;188(4):218.*

[148] Khan SA, Singh RK, Navit S, Chadha D, Johri N, Navit P, Sharma A, Bahuguna R. Relationship Between Dental Fluorosis and Intelligence Quotient of School Going Children In and Around Lucknow District: A Cross-Sectional Study. *J Clin Diagn Res. 2015 Nov;9(11):ZC10-5.*

[149] Sebastian ST, Sunitha S. A cross-sectional study to assess the intelligence quotient (IQ) of school going children aged 10-12 years in villages of Mysore district, India with different fluoride levels. *J Indian Soc Pedod Prev Dent. 2015 Oct-Dec;33(4):307-11.*

[150] Nagarajappa R, Pujara P, Sharda AJ, Asawa K, Tak M, Aapaliya P, Bhanushali N. Comparative Assessment of Intelligence Quotient among Children Living in High and Low Fluoride Areas of Kutch, India-a Pilot Study. *Iran J Public Health. 2013 Aug;42(8):813-8.*

[151] Seraj B, Shahrabi M, Shadfar M, Ahmadi R, Fallahzadeh M, Eslamlu HF, Kharazifard MJ. Effect of high water fluoride concentration on the intellectual development of children in makoo/iran. *J Dent (Tehran). 2012 Summer;9(3):221-9.*

[152] Starek-Świechowicz B, Starek A. [Ethylene glycol and propylene glycol ethers - Reproductive and developmental toxicity]. *Med Pr. 2015;66(5):725-37. Review. Polish.*

[153] Mai T, Rakhmatullina E, Bleek K, Boye S, Yuan J, Völkel A, Gräwert M, Cheaib Z, Eick S, Günter C, Lederer A, Lussi A, Taubert A. Poly(ethylene oxide)-b-poly(3-sulfopropyl methacrylate) block copolymers for calcium phosphate mineralization and biofilm inhibition. *Biomacromolecules. 2014 Nov 10;15(11):3901-14.*

[154] Andra SS, Makris KC. Thyroid disrupting chemicals in plastic additives and thyroid health. *J Environ Sci Health C Environ Carcinog Ecotoxicol Rev.2012;30(2):107-51.*

[155] Jenkinson HF. Beyond the oral microbiome. *Environ Microbiol. 2011 Dec;13(12):3077-87.*

[156] http://www.toxicteeth.org/natCamp_ADAresponds_haleyrebuttal.aspx

[157] Wilson G, Conway DI. Mouthwash use and associated head and neck cancer risk. *Evid Based Dent. 2016 Mar;17(1):8-9.*

[158] Friemel J, Foraita R, Günther K, Heibeck M, Günther F, Pflueger M, Pohlabeln H, Behrens T, Bullerdiek J, Nimzyk R, Ahrens W. Pretreatment oral hygiene habits and survival of head and neck squamous cell carcinoma (HNSCC) patients. *BMC Oral Health. 2016 Mar 11;16(1):33.*

[159] Sood P, Devi M A, Narang R, V S, Makkar DK. Comparative efficacy of oil pulling and chlorhexidine on oral malodor: a randomized controlled trial. *J Clin Diagn Res. 2014 Nov;8(11):ZC18-21.*

[160] Vlachojannis C, Al-Ahmad A, Hellwig E, Chrubasik S. Listerine® Products: An Update on the Efficacy and Safety. *Phytother Res. 2016 Mar;30(3):367-73.*

[161] Petersson J, Carlström M, Schreiber O, Phillipson M, Christoffersson G, Jägare A, Roos S, Jansson EA, Persson AE, Lundberg JO, Holm L. Gastroprotective and blood pressure lowering effects of dietary nitrate are abolished by an antiseptic mouthwash. *Free Radic Biol Med. 2009 Apr 15;46(8):1068-75.*

[162] Kapil V, Haydar SM, Pearl V, Lundberg JO, Weitzberg E, Ahluwalia A. Physiological role for nitrate-reducing oral bacteria in blood pressure control. *Free Radic Biol Med. 2013 Feb;55:93-100.*

[163] http://www.medicaldaily.com/antiseptic-mouthwash-raises-heart-attack-risk-blood-pressure-chlorhexidine-kills-good-bacteria-helps

[164] Lewington S., Clarke R., Qizilbash N., Peto R., Collins R., Collaboration P.S. Age-specific relevance of usual blood pressure to vascular mortality: a meta-analysis of individual data for one million adults in 61 prospective studies. *Lancet. 2002;360:1903–1913.*

[165] Chow AY, Hirsch GH, Buttar HS. Nephrotoxic and hepatotoxic effects of triclosan and chlorhexidine in rats. *Toxicol Appl Pharmacol. 1977 Oct;42(1):1-10.*

[166] Wright YL, Swartz, JM. *Secrets to Lose Toxic Belly Fat! Heal Your Sick Metabolism Using State-Of-The-Art Medical Testing and Treatment With Detoxification, Diet, Lifestyle, Supplements, and Bioidentical Hormones.* Lulu Press. 2012.

[167] Thornton-Evans G, Eke P, Wei L, Palmer A, Moeti R, Hutchins S, Borrell LN; Centers for Disease Control and Prevention (CDC). Periodontitis among adults aged≥30 years - United States, 2009-2010. *MMWR Surveill Summ. 2013 Nov 22;62 Suppl3:129-35.*

[168] Kassebaum NJ, Bernabé E, Dahiya M, Bhandari B, Murray CJ, Marcenes W. Global burden of severe periodontitis in 1990-2010: a systematic review and meta-regression. *J Dent Res. 2014 Nov;93(11):1045-53.*

[169] http://www1.umn.edu/perio/tobacco/tobperio.html

[170] Ahmed U, Tanwir F. Association of periodontal pathogenesis and cardiovascular diseases: a literature review. *Oral Health Prev Dent. 2015;13(1):21-7.*

[171] Casanova L, Hughes FJ, Preshaw PM. Diabetes and periodontal disease: a two-way relationship. *Br Dent J. 2014 Oct;217(8):433-7.*

[172] Varshney S, Gautam A. Poor periodontal health as a risk factor for development of pre-eclampsia in pregnant women. *J Indian Soc Periodontol. 2014 May;18(3):321-5.*

[173] Ziebolz D, Rost C, Schmidt J, Waldmann-Beushausen R, Schöndube FA, Mausberg RF, Danner BC.

Periodontal Bacterial DNA and Their Link to Human Cardiac Tissue: Findings of a Pilot Study. *Thorac Cardiovasc Surg. 2015 Oct 5.*

[174] Oliveira FA, Forte CP, Silva PG, Lopes CB, Montenegro RC, Santos ÂK, Sobrinho CR, Mota MR, Sousa FB, Alves AP. Molecular Analysis of Oral Bacteria in Heart Valve of Patients With Cardiovascular Disease by Real-Time Polymerase Chain Reaction. *Medicine (Baltimore). 2015 Nov;94(47):e2067.*

[175] Hosomi N, Aoki S, Matsuo K, Deguchi K, Masugata H, Murao K, Ichihara N, OhyamaH, Dobashi H, Nezu T, Ohtsuki T, Yasuda O, Soejima H, Ogawa H, Izumi Y, Kohno M, Tanaka J, Matsumoto M. Association of serum antiperiodontal pathogen antibody with ischemic stroke. *Cerebrovasc Dis. 2012;34(5-6):385-92.*

[176] Kumar M, Mishra L, Mohanty R, Nayak R. "Diabetes and gum disease: the diabolic duo". *Diabetes Metab Syndr. 2014 Oct-Dec;8(4):255-8.*

[177] Marchesan JT, Gerow EA, Schaff R, Taut AD, Shin SY, Sugai J, Brand D, Burberry A, Jorns J, Lundy SK, Nuñez G, Fox DA, Giannobile WV. Porphyromonas gingivalis oral infection exacerbates the development and severity of collagen-induced arthritis. *Arthritis Res Ther. 2013 Nov 12;15(6):R186.*

[178] Meisel P, Holtfreter B, Biffar R, Suemnig W, Kocher T. Association of periodontitis with the risk of oral leukoplakia. *Oral Oncol. 2012 Sep;48(9):859-63.*

[179] Macedo JF, Ribeiro RA, Machado FC, Assis NM, Alves RT, Oliveira AS, Ribeiro LC. Periodontal disease and oral health-related behavior as factors associated with preterm birth: a case-control study in south-eastern Brazil. *J Periodontal Res. 2014 Aug;49(4):458-64.*

[180] Kennedy, D. *How to Save Your Teeth. Toxic-Free Preventative Dentistry.* U.S.A. David C. Kennedy. 1993.

[181] Sepúlveda B. Amebiasis: host-pathogen biology. *Rev Infect Dis. 1982 Nov-Dec;4(6):1247-53. Review.*

[182] Wright YL, Swartz, JM. *Secrets to Lose Toxic Belly Fat! Heal Your Sick Metabolism Using State-Of-The-Art Medical Testing and Treatment With Detoxification, Diet, Lifestyle, Supplements, and Bioidentical Hormones.* Lulu Press. 2012.

[183] Horie N, Kawano R, Kaneko T, Shimoyama T. Methotrexate-related lymphoproliferative disorder arising in the gingiva of a patient with rheumatoid arthritis. *Aust Dent J. 2015 Sep;60(3):408-11.*

[184] Montevecchi M, Dorigo A, Cricca M, Checchi L. Comparison of the antibacterial activity of an ozonated oil with chlorhexidine digluconate and povidone-iodine. A disk diffusion test. *New Microbiol. 2013 Jul;36(3):289-302.*

[185] Patel PV, Patel A, Kumar S, Holmes JC. Effect of subgingival application of topical ozonated olive oil in the treatment of chronic periodontitis: a randomized, controlled, double blind, clinical and microbiological study. *Minerva Stomatol. 2012 Sep;61(9):381-98.*

[186] Patel PV, Kumar S, Vidya GD, Patel A, Holmes JC, Kumar V. Cytological assessment of healing palatal donor site wounds and grafted gingival wounds after application of ozonated oil: an eighteen-month randomized controlled clinical trial. *Acta Cytol. 2012;56(3):277-84.*

[187] Patel PV, Patel A, Kumar S, Holmes JC. Evaluation of ozonated olive oil with or without adjunctive application of calcium sodium phosphosilicate on post-surgical root dentin hypersensitivity: a randomized, double-blinded, controlled, clinical trial. *Minerva Stomatol. 2013 May;62(5):147-61*

[188] Huggins HA, Levy TE. *Uninformed consent. The hidden dangers in dental care.* Hampton Roads Publishing Company. Charlottesville, VA. 1999.

[189] Huggins, H. *Uninformed Consent.* . Hapton Roads Publishing Company, Inc. Charlottesville, Va. 1999 P.86.

[190] Pessi T, Karhunen V, Karjalainen PP, Ylitalo A, Airaksinen JK, Niemi M,Pietila M, Lounatmaa K, Haapaniemi T, Lehtimäki T, Laaksonen R, Karhunen PJ,Mikkelsson J. Bacterial signatures in thrombus aspirates of patients with myocardial infarction. *Circulation. 2013 Mar 19;127(11):1219-28, e1-6.*

[191] Joshipura KJ, Pitiphat W, Hung HC, Willett WC, Colditz GA, Douglass CW. Pulpal inflammation and incidence of coronary heart disease. *J Endod. 2006 Feb;32(2):99-103.*

[192] Breebaart AC, Bijlsma JW, van Eden W. 16-year remission of rheumatoid arthritis after unusually

vigorous treatment of closed dental foci. *Clin Exp Rheumatol. 2002 Jul-Aug;20(4):555-7.*
[193] http://www.westonaprice.org/
[194] Price, W. *Dental Infections Oral and Systemic.* Penton Press Co., Cleveland, OH. 1923.
[195] Dodd RB, Dodds RN, Hocomb JB.An endodontically induced maxillary sinusitis.*J Endod.1984 Oct;10(10):504-6.*
[196] Fava LR. Calcium hydroxide paste in the maxillary sinus: a case report. *Int Endod J. 1993 Sep;26(5):306-10.*
[197] Kaplowitz GJ. Penetration of the maxillary sinus by overextended gutta percha cones. Report of two cases. *Clin Prev Dent. 1985 Mar-Apr;7(2):28-30.*
[198] Kobayashi A. Asymptomatic aspergillosis of the maxillary sinus associated with foreign body of endodontic origin. Report of a case. *Int J Oral Maxillofac Surg. 1995 Jun;24(3):243-4.*
[199] Ehrich DG, Brian JD Jr, Walker WA. Sodium hypochlorite accident: inadvertent injection into the maxillary sinus. *J Endod. 1993 Apr;19(4):180-2.*
[200] Pashley DH. Dentin-predentin complex and its permeability: physiologic overview. *J Dent Res. 1985 Apr;64 Spec No:613-20.*
[201] Gatot A, Arbelle J, Leiberman A, Yanai-Inbar I. Effects of sodium hypochlorite on soft tissues after its inadvertent injection beyond the root apex. *J Endod. 1991 Nov;17(11):573-4. Review.*
[202] Gatot A, Arbelle J, Leiberman A, Yanai-Inbar I. Effects of sodium hypochlorite on soft tissues after its inadvertent injection beyond the root apex. *J Endod. 1991 Nov;17(11):573-4. Review.*
[203] Reeh ES, Messer HH. Long-term paresthesia following inadvertent forcing of sodium hypochlorite through perforation in maxillary incisor. *Endod Dent Traumatol. 1989 Aug;5(4):200-3.*
[204] Fouad AF, Krell KV, McKendry DJ, Koorbusch GF, Olson RA. Clinical evaluation of five electronic root canal length measuring instruments. *J Endod. 1990 Sep;16(9):446-9.*
[205] Fairbourn DR, McWalter GM, Montgomery S. The effect of four preparation techniques on the amount of apically extruded debris. *J Endod. 1987 Mar;13(3):102-8.*
[206] Engstrom B, Frostell G. Experiences of bacteriological root canal control. *Acta Odontol Scand. 1964 Feb;22:43-69.*
[207] Harris WE. Conservative treatment of a large radicular cyst: report of case. *J Am Dent Assoc. 1971 Jun;82(6):1390-4.*
[208] Bouquot JE, LaMarche MG: Ischemic Osteonecrosis under fixed partial denture pontics: Radiographic and microscopic features in 38 patients with chronic pain. *J Prosthetic Dent 81: 148-158.*
[209] Marx, R.E. *Oral and Intravenous bisphosphonate-induced osteonecrosis of the jaws.* Chicago: Quintessence. 2011: 11-12.
[210] Marx RE, Swatari Y, Fortin M, Broumand V. Bisphophonate-induce exposed bone (osteonecrosis/osteopetrosis) of the jaws: Risk factors, recognition, prevention, and treatment. *J Oral Maxillofac Surg 2005;63: 1567-1575.*
[211] Ruggiero SL, Dodson TB, Assael LA, Landesberg R, Marx RE, Mehotra B (Task Force on Bisphophonate-Related Osteonecrosis of the Jaws, American Association of Oral and Maxillofacial Surgeons). American Association of Oral and Maxillofacial Surgeons position pater on bisphosphonate-related osteonecrosis of the jaw-2009 update. *Aust Endod J 2009; 35:119-130.*
[212] Vidal-Real C, Pérez-Sayáns M, Suárez-Peñaranda JM, Gándara-Rey JM, García-García A. Osteonecrosis of the jaws in 194 patients who have undergone intravenous bisphosphonate therapy in Spain. *Med Oral Patol Oral Cir Bucal. 2015 May 1;20(3):e267-72.*
[213] Ripamonti, CI, Maniezzo M, Pessi, MA, Boldini, S. Treatment of osteonecrosis of the jaw (ONJ) by medical ozone gas insufflation. A case report. *Tumori 2012. May-June; 98(3): 72-75.*
[214] Cole, G. Treatment of bisphosphonate related osteonecrosis of the jaw (BRONJ) with oxygen-ozone therapy: a case report. *J of Implant and Advanced Clinical Dentistry, Vol 5, No. 5, May 2013.*
[215] Marx, R.E. *Oral and Intravenous bisphosphonate-induced osteonecrosis of the jaws.* Chicago:

Quintessence. 2011: 59-66.

[216] Cole, G. Treatment of bisphosphonate related osteonecrosis of the jaw (BRONJ) with oxygen-ozone therapy: a case report. *J of Implant and Advanced Clinical Dentistry, Vol 5, No. 5, May 2013.*

[217] Agrillo, A et al. Bisphosphonate-related osteonecrosis of the jaw (BRONJ): five year experience in the treatment of 131 cases with ozone therapy. *Eur Rev Med Pharmacol Sci. 2012 Nov;16(2): 1741-1747.*

[218] Hamadeh IS, Ngwa BA, Gong Y. Drug induced osteonecrosis of the jaw. *Cancer Treat Rev. 2015 May;41(5):455-64.*

[219] Rustemeyer J, Melenberg A, Junker K, Sari-Rieger A. Osteonecrosis of the maxilla related to long-standing methamphetamine abuse: a possible new aspect in the etiology of osteonecrosis of the jaw. *Oral Maxillofac Surg. 2014 Jun;18(2):237-41.*

[220] Bick RL: *Disorders of Thrombosis and Hemostasis. Clinical and Laboratory Practice.* Roger Bick (ed). Third ed., Philadelphia, PA: Lippincott Williams and Williams; 2002

[221] Brown P, Cran L: Avascular necrosis of bone in patients with human immunodeficiency virus infection: report of 6 cases and review of the literature. *Clinical Infectious Diseases 2001; 32:1221-1226.*

[222] Gandhi YR, Pal US, Singh N. Neuralgia-inducing cavitational osteonecrosis in a patient seeking dental implants. *Natl J Maxillofac Surg. 2012 Jan;3(1):84-6.*

[223] Haley B. Characterization and identification of chemical toxicants isolated from cavitational material and infected root canalled teeth; in situ testing of teeth for toxicity and infection; Proceedings of Annual meeting, *International Academy of Oral medicine and Toxicology; San Diego, California; 1997.*

[224] Bouquot JE, Roberts AM, Person P, Christian J. Neuralgia-inducing cavitational osteonecrosis (NICO). Osteomyelitis in 224 jawbone samples from patients with facial neuralgia. *Oral Surg Oral Med Oral Pathol. 1992 Mar;73(3):307-19; discussion 319-20. Review.*

[225] Bouquot JE: Characterization and identification of chemical toxicants isolated from cavitational material and infected root canalled teeth; in situ testing of teeth for toxicity and infection. *Proceedings of Annual Meeting, International Academy of Oral Medicine and Toxicology; San Diego, CA; 1997.*

[226] Lechner J, VonBaehr V. Rantes and fibroblast growth factor in jawbone cavitations; Triggers for systemic disease? *International Journal of Medicine 2013: 6, 277-290.*

[227] Lechner J. Chronic osteonecrosis of jawbone (NICO): Unknown trigger for systemic disease and a possible new integrative approach? *J Altern Med Res 2013;5(3):243-250.*

[228] Lechner J., von Baehr V. Hyperactive signaling pathways of chemokine RANTES/CCL5 in osteopathies of jawbone in breast cancer patients—case report and research. *Breast Cancer: Basic and Clinical Research 2014: 8, 89-96.*

[229] Campisi G, Fedele S, Fusco V, Pizzo G, Di Fede O, Bedogni A. Epidemiology,clinical manifestations, risk reduction and treatment strategies of jaw osteonecrosis in cancer patients exposed to antiresorptive agents. *Future Oncol. 2014 Feb;10(2):257-75.*

[230] Lechner J, von Baehr V. RANTES and fibroblast growth factor 2 in jawbone cavitations: triggers for systemic disease? *Int J Gen Med. 2013 Apr 22;6:277-90.*

[231] Black A., *G. V. Black's Work on Operative Dentistry, vol. 1.* Chicago: Medico-Dental Publishing Company, 1936, p. 4.

[232] Bouquot JE, Christian J. Long-term effects of jawbone curettage on the pain of facial neuralgia. *J Oral Maxillofac Surg. 1995 Apr;53(4):387-97; discussion 397-9.*

[233] Lechner J, Mayer W. Immune messengers in neuralgia inducing cavitational osteonecrosis (NICO) in jawbone and systemic interference. *European Journal of Integrative Medicine. 2 (2010) 71-77.*

[234] Bouquot JE, Roberts, AM, Person P: Neuralgia-inducing Cavitational Osteonecrosis (NICO): Osteomyelitis in 224 jawbone samples from patients with facial neuralgias. *Oral Surg Oral Med Oral Pathol 1992; 73: 307-319.*

[235] Barrett WC: *Oral Pathology and Practice.* Philadelphia, PA, S.S. White Dental Mfg. Co, 1898.

[236] Noel HR: A lecture on caries and necrosis of bone. *Am J Dent Sci (series 3):189, 1868.*

[237] Black GV: *A work on special dental pathology.* Chicago: Medico-Dental Co, 1915; 388-391.

[238] Neville BW, Damm DD, Allen CM, Bouquot JE. *Oral and Maxillofacial Pathology.* Philadelphia: WB Saunders Co; 2009: 866-869.
[239] Haley B. Characterization and identification of chemical toxicants isolated from cavitational material and infected root canalled teeth; in situ testing of teeth for toxicity and infection. *Proceedings of Annual meeting, International Academy of Oral medicine and Toxicology; San Diego, California; 1997.*
[240] Shankland WE 2nd. Medullary and odontogenic disease in the painful jaw: clinicopathologic review of 500 consecutive lesions. *Cranio. 2002 Oct;20(4):295-303.*
[241] Ratner EJ, Person P, Kleinman DJ, Shklar G, Socranksy SS: Jawbone cavities and trigeminal and atypical facial neuralgias. *Oral Surg 19790, 48, no. 1: 3-20.*
[242] Bouquot JE, Roberts AM, Person P: Neuralgia-inducing cavitational Osteonecrosis (NICO): Osteomyelitis in 224 jawbone samples from patients with facial neuralgias. *Oral Surg Oral Med Oral Pathol 1992; 73: 312-315.*
[243] Bouquot JE, Roberts AM, Person P, Christian J. Neuralgia-inducing cavitational osteonecrosis (NICO). Osteomyelitis in 224 jawbone samples from patients with facial neuralgias. *Oral Surg Oral Med Oral Pathol. 1992 Mar;73(3):307-19;discussion 319-20. Review.*
[244] Ratner EJ, Person P, Kleinman DJ, Shklar G, Socransky SS. Jawbone cavities and trigeminal and atypical facial neuralgias. *Oral Surg Oral Med Oral Pathol. 1979 Jul;48(1):3-20.*
[245] Brotóns A, Peñarrocha M. Orofacial neurogenic pain and maxillofacial ischemic osteonecrosis. A review. *Med Oral. 2003 May-Jul;8(3):157-65.*
[246] Gandhi YR, Pal US, Singh N. Neuralgia-inducing cavitational osteonecrosis in a patient seeking dental implants. *Natl J Maxillofac Surg. 2012 Jan;3(1):84-6.*
[247] http://whale.to/d/cavitations.html
[248] Bouquot JE, Christian J. Long-term effects of jawbone curettage on the pain of facial neuralgia. *J Oral Maxillofac Surg. 1995 Apr;53(4):387-97; discussion 397-9.*
[249] Rehme M. *Unexplained Dental Pain Explained:Tooth Extractions, Cavitations and the Periodontal Ligament* 2014. www.toothbody.com.
[250] http://whale.to/d/cavitations.html
[251] http://www.mgoldmandds.com/Cavitations.htm
[252] http://www.lovingourguts.com/cavitation-surgery-my-experience/
[253] http://www.livingnetwork.co.za/dentalnetwork/cavitations/my-cavitation-cleaning-experience/
[254] Bouquot JE, LaMarche MG: Ischemic Osteonecrosis under fixed partial denture pontics: Radiographic and microscopic features in 38 patients with chronic pain. *J Prosthetic Dent 81: 148-158.*
[255] http://www.mgoldmandds.com/Cavitations.htm
[256] Hauser F, Gaydarov N, Badoud I, Vazquez L, Bernard JP, Ammann P. Clinical and histological evaluation of postextraction platelet-rich fibrin socket filling: a prospective randomized controlled study. *Implant Dent. 2013 Jun;22(3):295-303.*
[257] Ratner EJ, Person P, Kleinman DJ, et al: Jawbone cavities and trigeminal and atypical facial neuralgias. *Oral Surg Oral Med Oral Pathol 1079; 48, mo. 1: 3-20.*
[258] Imbeau J: Introduction to Through-Transmission Alveolar Ultrasonography (TAU) in Dental Medicine. *Cranio April 2005, Vol. 23, No.2: 100-112.*
[259] Bedogni A, Fedele S, Bedogni G, Scoletta M, Favia G, Colella G, Agrillo A, Bettini G, Di Fede O, Oteri G, Fusco V, Gabriele M, Ottolenghi L, Valsecchi S,Porter S, Petruzzi M, Arduino P, D'Amato S, Ungari C, Fung Polly PL, Saia G, Campisi G. Staging of osteonecrosis of the jaw requires computed tomography for accurate definition of the extent of bony disease. *Br J Oral Maxillofac Surg.2014 Sep;52(7):603-8.*
[260] Esposito SA, et al. A Novel Method to Estimate the Volume of Bone Defects Using Cone-Beam Computer Tomography; an In Vitro Study. *JOE 2013 Sept; 39(9): 1111-1115.*
[261] M. Joujeim, T.J. Prihoda, et al. Evaluation of high-resolution cone-beam computed tomography in the

detection of simulated inter-radicular bone lesions. *Dentomaxillofacial Radiology (2009) 38, 156-162.*
[262] B. Felipe, et al. Comparison between cone-beam and multi-slice computed tomography for identification of simulated bone lesions. *Braz. oral res. [online].* 2011, vol.25, n.4, pp. 362-368. ISSN 1806-8324.
[263] Tyndall DA, Rathore S. Cone-Beam CT Diagnostic Applications: Caries, Periodontal Bone Assessment, and Endodontic Applications. *Dent Clin N Am 52 (2008) 825-841.*
[264] Patil NA, Gadda R, Salvi R. Cone Beam Computed Tomography: Adding the Third Dimension. *J Contemp Dent 2012;2(3):84-88*
[265] Cohen S: Diagnostic procedures. In: *Pathways of the pulp. 6$^{th}$ ed.* Cohen S. Burns RC (eds). St. Louis: CV Mosby Co; 1994:10.
[266] Shankland W. *Differential Diagnosis of NICO Lesions.* TMJ & Facial Pain Center Columbus, OH.
[267] L. He, Y. Lin, X. Hu, Y. Zhang, and J. We, "A comparative study of platelet-rich fibrin (PRF) and platelet-rich plasma (PRP) on the effect of proliferation and differentiation of rat osteoblasts in vitro." *Oral Surg Oral Med Oral Pathol Oral Radiol Endod. 2009 Nov;108(5):707-13.*
[268] Thorat M, Pradeep AR, Pallavi B. Clinical effect of autologous platelet-rich fibrin in the treatment of intra-bony defects: a controlled clinical trial. *J Clin Periodontol. 2011 Oct;38(10):925-32.*
[269] Dohan DM, Choukroun J, Diss A, Dohan SL, Dohan AJ, Mouhyi J, Gogly B. Platelet-rich fibrin (PRF): a second-generation platelet concentrate. Part I: technological concepts and evolution. *Oral Surg Oral Med Oral Pathol Oral Radiol Endod. 2006 Mar;101(3):e37-44.*
[270] J.M. Karp, F. Sarraf, M.S. Shoichet, and Davies, J.E. Fibrin filled scaffolds for bones-tissue engineering: an in vivo study. *Journal of Biomedical Materials Research A, vol. 71, no. 1, pp. 162-171, 2004.*
[271] D.M.S. Ehrenfest, G. M. de Peppo, P. Doglioli, and G. Sammartino. Slow release of growth factors and thrombospondin-1 in Choukroun's platelet-rich fibrin (PRF): a gold standard to achieve for all surgical platelet concentrates technologies. *Growth Factors, vol. 27, no. 1, pp. 63-69, 2009.*
[272] Bouquot JE, Christian J. Long-term effects of jawbone curettage on the pain of facial neuralgia. *J Oral Maxillofac Surg. 1995 Apr;53(4):387-97; discussion 397-9.*
[273] Gates D. *The Body Ecology Diet: Recovering Your Health and Rebuilding Your Immunity.* Hay House, Inc. Carlsbad, CA. 2011.
[274] https://iaomt.org
[275] http://www.hugginsappliedhealing.com
[276] El Hadary AA, Yassin HH, Mekhemer ST, Holmes JC, Grootveld M. Evaluation of the effect of ozonated plant oils on the quality of osseointegration of dental implants under the influence of Cyclosporin A an in vivo study. *J Oral Implantol.2011 Apr;37(2):247-57.*
[277] https://www.hugginsappliedhealing.com/faqs.php
[278] http://www.hugginsappliedhealing.com/faqs.php
[279] T.E.R.F. Toxic elements research foundation discovers hidden dangers within dental implants. *D-D Media Implant.*
[280] http://www.melisa.org/contact-us/melisa-laboratories/
[281] Oshima M, Tsuji T. Whole Tooth Regeneration as a Future Dental Treatment. *Adv Exp Med Biol. 2015;881:255-69.*
[282] Sun HH, Jin T, Yu Q, Chen FM. Biological approaches toward dental pulp regeneration by tissue engineering. *J Tissue Eng Regen Med. 2011 Apr;5(4):e1-16.*
[283] Yuan Z, Nie H, Wang S, Lee CH, Li A, Fu SY, Zhou H, Chen L, Mao JJ. Biomaterial selection for tooth regeneration. *Tissue Eng Part B Rev. 2011 Oct;17(5):373-88. Review.*
[284] http://www.apha.org/policies-and-advocacy/public-health-policy-statements/policy-database/2014/07/24/14/29/opposition-to-prophylactic-removal-of-third-molars-wisdom-teeth
[285] Huggins H. Blood and DNA data show dental materials can create autoimmune diseases. *Dental Materials News Release (1.0).*

[286] T.E.R.F. Little understood dental condition provides clues to the source for many of today's deadly diseases. *D-Day Media Cav.*
[287] Polydorou O, Pelz K, Hahn P. Antibacterial effect of an ozone device and its comparison with two dentin-bonding systems. *Eur J Oral Sci. 2006 Aug;114(4):349-53.*
[288] Intahphuak S, Khonsung P, Panthong A. Anti-inflammatory, analgesic, and antipyretic activities of virgin coconut oil. *Pharm Biol. 2010 Feb;48(2):151-7.*
[289] Singh A, Purohit B. Tooth brushing, oil pulling and tissue regeneration: A review of holistic approaches to oral health. *J Ayurveda Integr Med. 2011 Apr;2(2):64-8.*
[290] Asokan S, Rathan J, Muthu MS, Rathna PV, Emmadi P; Raghuraman; Chamundeswari. Effect of oil pulling on Streptococcus mutans count in plaque and saliva using Dentocult SM Strip mutans test: a randomized, controlled, triple-blind study. *J Indian Soc Pedod Prev Dent. 2008 Mar;26(1):12-7.*
[291] Kaushik M, Reddy P, Sharma R, Udameshi P, Mehra N, Marwaha A. The Effect of Coconut Oil pulling on Streptococcus mutans Count in Saliva in Comparison with Chlorhexidine Mouthwash. *J Contemp Dent Pract. 2016 Jan 1;17(1):38-41.*
[292] Asokan S, Emmadi P, Chamundeswari R. Effect of oil pulling on plaque induced gingivitis: a randomized, controlled, triple-blind study. *Indian J Dent Res. 2009 Jan-Mar;20(1):47-51.*
[293] Sood P, Devi M A, Narang R, V S, Makkar DK. Comparative efficacy of oil pulling and chlorhexidine on oral malodor: a randomized controlled trial. *J Clin Diagn Res. 2014 Nov;8(11):ZC18-21.*
[294] Asokan S, Kumar RS, Emmadi P, Raghuraman R, Sivakumar N. Effect of oil pulling on halitosis and microorganisms causing halitosis: a randomized controlled pilot trial. *J Indian Soc Pedod Prev Dent. 2011 Apr-Jun;29(2):90-4.*
[295] Peedikayil FC, Sreenivasan P, Narayanan A. Effect of coconut oil in plaque related gingivitis - A preliminary report. *Niger Med J. 2015 Mar-Apr;56(2):143-7.*
[296] Asokan S, Rathan J, Muthu MS, Rathna PV, Emmadi P; Raghuraman; Chamundeswari. Effect of oil pulling on Streptococcus mutans count in plaque and saliva usingDentocult SM Strip mutans test: a randomized, controlled, triple-blind study. *J Indian Soc Pedod Prev Dent. 2008 Mar;26(1):12-7.*
[297] Schuppan D, Pickert G, Ashfaq-Khan M, Zevallos V. Non-celiac wheat sensitivity: differential diagnosis, triggers and implications. *Best Pract Res Clin Gastroenterol. 2015 Jun;29(3):469-76.*
[298] de Lorgeril M, Salen P. Gluten and wheat intolerance today: are modern wheat strains involved? *Int J Food Sci Nutr. 2014 Aug;65(5):577-81.*
[299] Mansueto P, D'Alcamo A, Seidita A, Carroccio A. Food allergy in irritable bowel syndrome: The case of non-celiac wheat sensitivity. *World J Gastroenterol. 2015 Jun 21;21(23):7089-109.*
[300] Carroccio A, D'Alcamo A, Cavataio F, Soresi M, Seidita A, Sciumè C, Geraci G, Iacono G, Mansueto P. High Proportions of People With Nonceliac Wheat Sensitivity Have Autoimmune Disease or Antinuclear Antibodies. *Gastroenterology. 2015Sep;149(3):596-603.e1.*
[301] Chaudhari LK, Jawale BA, Sharma S, Sharma H, Kumar CD, Kulkarni PA. Antimicrobial activity of commercially available essential oils against Streptococcus mutans. *J Contemp Dent Pract. 2012 Jan 1;13(1):71-4*

Made in the USA
Columbia, SC
21 November 2023

26863499R00055